THE BELOW
TEN THOUSAND
WAY

This is an IndieMosh book
brought to you by MoshPit Publishing
an imprint of Mosher's Business Support Pty Ltd
PO Box 147
Hazelbrook NSW 2779
indiemosh.com.au

Cataloguing-in-Publication entry is available from the National Library of Australia: http://catalogue.nla.gov.au/

Title: The Below Ten Thousand Way to a clinician-led safety culture

Author: Smith, Pete (1963–)

ISBNs: 978-1-925959-24-6 (paperback)
           978-1-925959-25-3 (ebook – epub)
           978-1-925959-26-0 (ebook – mobi)

Subjects: Medical: Nursing Fundamentals & Skills; Anesthesia; Anesthesiology; Social, Ethical & Legal Issues

Cover design by Pete Smith

Cover layout by Ally Mosher at allymosher.com

Kimguard blue fabric image from Adobe Stock. Other cover images copyright © Pete Smith 2019

*If you are a patient
and you are going to the operating theatre,
buy a copy of this book
and put it under your theatre trolley.*

*Chances are, if the staff know
what's in this book,
you will have a shorter, safer procedure
with less chance of a surgical site infection.*

Pete's mum

THE **BELOW TEN THOUSAND** WAY

to a clinician-led safety culture

A BEGINNER'S HANDBOOK

PETE SMITH

DEDICATIONS

For their gift of inspiration, high advocacy and strong identity within the healthcare system I would like to dedicate this book to

Dr Patricia Nicholson
and
Sally Sutherland-Fraser

two nurses who were obliged to deliver the Judith Cornell Oration for ACORN (Australian College of Operating Room Nurses) and whom, in turn, spoke about outliers as the key to success and the question of self-identity or what it means to identify as a nurse.

In doing so Patricia and Sally perfectly described the key challenges in our clinician-led culture change and thus our 'Below Ten Thousand' journey.

Many thanks for your impassioned sharing.

CONTENTS

Dedications ix

Introduction... xv
   Lived Experience... xvii

Below Ten Thousand..1
   Profiles... 3
      John..3
      Pete 3
      Suzanne 4
      Tim 4
      Gaye 4
      Rob..5
      Ash..5
   A Short History of Below Ten Thousand 6

Towards a Compassionate Safety Culture 9
   Working intelligently with compassion 11
   Why clinician-led culture change? 13
   Twenty-five words or less 17
   Best Practice... 19
      Best Practice and Below Ten Thousand 19
      The 'Reasonable Person' Test.............................. 23
   Principles of Below Ten Thousand...................... 24
   Clinician-Led Culture Change 27
      A worthwhile challenge.................................... 27
   The half-life of medical knowledge 30

Collaboration 31
   High Performance Teams?.................................. 33
   A Hosed Down Hierarchy 35

Engagement 38
    Relationship Building 39
    Formal Presentations 39
    Signage 40
    Pamphlets 40
    Orientation 40
    Measurement 41
    On-selling 41
    Further potential 42

An Unfolding Story 45
    All for one and one for all 47
    Further Research Required 48
    Dickensian culture 49
    Rogues of Safety 52

Plan; Do; Check; Build 55
    Phase 1 55
    Phase 2 56
    Phase 3 60

'Within and as a team' 63

Flawless Teams 66
    Trust 67
    Bullying as a distraction 67

Work Flow and Intensification 71

Creating Flowing Work Designs 73
    Next Step Thinking and Unc0mpl3xity Theory 73
    Logic Process 78
    Developing new pathways 82

Human Factors 85
    Plan 87
    Assembling the Core Emergency Team 88

Team Fluxing 93

Work intensification 96

Tectonic Plate Tetris Theory of Workload............. 96

Fatigue..103

Fatigue...105

The Edge of Coping 105

Fatigue as a Workplace Injury (FAWPI).............125

How to use FAWPI 126

IM SAFE...129

Summation: The Below Ten Thousand Way to
Clinician-led culture change.................................131

Rob's Top Ten Further Reading................................ 133

Advocacy 145

About the Author 148

INTRODUCTION

There is no place in healthcare that epitomises the notion of 'team' more than the operating theatre. If you asked anyone who works in one they would implore: 'Of course we are a team. We are all working with a common purpose towards a common goal.'

In fact, operating theatres are teams within teams, all working with a common purpose towards a common goal.

But how high a performance team are we?

Can we say we are a high performance team simply because we perform the miracle that is surgery every day?

Can we say we are a high performance team when bullying and incivility are common themes in interpersonal dynamics every day?

Can we say we are a high performance team when we push people to the very edge of their coping, and yet expect them to be perfect every day?

And can we say we are a high performance team when distraction, noise and obstacles are an endemic feature of every day?

The Below Ten Thousand Way is about creating high performance teams. As a ridiculously simple concept, it is the first step towards reconstructing behavioural and systemic processes that build an improved operating theatre performance environment.

It begins with just three words created by John Gibbs and myself, two Australian nurses with thirty years experience each in the perioperative clinical environment.

Those three words are 'Below Ten Thousand' and together they herald a smarter, safer, better dawn.

They usher in an era where team performance becomes more effective, harm free, and less exhausting.

They provide a framework where existential challenges and fear are replaced by a sustainable robustness within which ordinary people may perform well in an excellent system of work.

John and I chose to disrupt the expectation that operating theatre staff should be able to achieve perfection despite an environment of overwhelming chaos and adversity.

In short, we simply sought to optimise the way we do the things we do but with realistic expectations and in so doing, we would give the nurses of the future a voice.

It began with three words which called for situational awareness and focus centred around the highly important task of caring for a patient.

Welcome to the operating theatre of the Below Ten Thousand age.

Pete Smith
July 2019

LIVED EXPERIENCE

I worked with a new graduate nurse not so long ago.

I asked her how she enjoyed her time in the operating theatres.

She said:

> *Each day depends on who I'm working with.*
> *Some days are good.*
> *Some days are horrible.*

We are all familiar with that sentiment.

And yet, we still think of ourselves strongly as a 'team'.

BELOW
TEN THOUSAND

PROFILES

JOHN

John Gibbs: The Guru. It was John's innovative thinking that led him to arrive at the answer to the problem of noise and distraction in the operating theatre.

Whilst the problem was being discussed at the global level, all proponents stopped thinking too soon. They stopped thinking when they had adequately outlined the problem.

It was John's genius that went that extra step and did what all great people do:

He reimagined the future and engineered a workable solution.

PETE

Pete Smith is me. I am simply the guerrilla in the room. All I did was refuse to let the idea die.

Following our discussion in Recovery one day whilst waiting for our next patients to arrive, John told me his solution to a problem we were both familiar with. Together we reverse engineered the steps necessary to bring John's idea to fruition.

We developed the 'Plan; Do; Check; Build' framework which provided the architecture we needed in order to fully collaborate with our peers, and we set to work.

Despite the excellent engagement of most of our peers, I take full responsibility for setting us on the path of rebellion when department managers failed us.

It was at that moment, when the need to find other avenues in order to progress our idea became necessary, that our clinician-led culture change effort through guerrilla marketing was born.

SUZANNE

Suzanne Rogan-Salifia is incredible. From the moment she heard our presentation at the ASPAAN Conference in Sydney, Suzanne was determined to introduce Below Ten Thousand at Liverpool Hospital where she is an educator.

Following a lot of hard work she introduced the concept to not just her own hospital, but to theatre suites across her entire Local Health District.

Suzanne is a vibrant safety culture advocate.

'Impressive' would be an appropriate description.

TIM

Dr Tim Leeuwenberg is a doctor on Kangaroo Island.

Tim is also a passionate and enthusiastic advocate for FOAMeD (Free Open Access Meducation) and SMACC (Social Media and Critical Care).

Tim enjoys a worldwide reputation for excellence in emergency care, so when Tim contacted John about taking the Below Ten Thousand idea to the SMACC Conference in Chicago, we were excited and delighted!

Tim, an amazing man of many talents and much energy, is responsible for encouraging us on our arduous journey.

GAYE

Gaye Coles is our own home-grown local champion.

Gaye has always loved and supported our Below Ten Thousand model.

We gave her Twinings Australian Afternoon Tea bags and pamphlets to take to the ICPAN Conference in Copenhagen. Somehow, in the course of her advocacy, she got to meet the Mayor of Copenhagen.

ROB

Rob Tomlinson is a true champion. 'Collaboration' is his middle name, and he doesn't mind taking 'no' for an answer, so long as it's not your final offer.

Rob truly moved heaven and earth to make Below Ten Thousand happen in hospitals throughout the UK.

A loyal Blackburn Rovers supporter, I don't think the word 'fear' is in his vocabulary, although the words 'Around, over or through,' are.

His gift for communication dissipates most obstacles.

ASH

Ash Kirk is a smart and determined quiet achiever.

When the going got tough, he recruited a steering committee to introduce Below Ten Thousand to his operating theatre at the Mercy Hospital, Dunedin, New Zealand.

But he didn't stop there.

Ash went on a journey of his own, delivering conference presentations and producing a video. He even brought the Haka to Below Ten Thousand and for that we are eternally grateful!

Steadfast and reliable, he accomplishes all without any fuss. You could say his motto is: 'Just do it!'

A SHORT HISTORY OF BELOW TEN THOUSAND

2013

- Idea conception
- Plan; Do; Check; Build process begins
- Awaiting approval from theatre managers; approval never eventuates
- Decision to progress as clinician-led culture change
- Guerrilla marketing campaign begins
- First presentation to Surgical Services Committee, Barwon Health

2014

- First presentation to Anaesthetic Department, Barwon Health
- Website started
- National ACORN Conference presentation, Melbourne
- State VPNG Conference presentation, Melbourne

2015

- ASPAAN Conference, Sydney
- Suzanne starts Below Ten Thousand at Liverpool Hospital, Sydney, and is nominated for a quality award

2016

- ACORN Conference presentation, Hobart

2017

- Rob starts work on Below Ten Thousand at East Lancashire Hospital Trust, UK, and produces a ground-breaking educational video

2018

- Ash starts Below Ten Thousand at Dunedin Mercy, New Zealand
- Rob wins a national Patient Safety Learning Award
- Ash and his team win the Catherine Scully Patient Safety Award

2019

- Below Ten Thousand is included in a 58 page UK Care Quality Commission report entitled 'Opening the door to change: NHS safety culture and the need for transformation'

TOWARDS A
COMPASSIONATE
SAFETY CULTURE

WORKING INTELLIGENTLY
WITH COMPASSION

Compassion is the clinician's calling card. Compassion is what leads us into our career. The potential for receiving compassion is what leads patients to our door when poor physical or mental health descends upon them.

Compassion keeps us but one step from barbarism.

If clinicians are by definition and identity compassionate, then the systems of work we engage in must possess an underlying architecture that permits that compassion.

Those who create our systems of work must be literate in compassionate design and must privilege human factors in order for clinicians to be able to perform that compassion effectively.

Compassion becomes the ultimate safety zone.

Compassion is what keeps healthcare a sanctuary for vulnerable people in need.

Erode compassion, demoralise the compassionate, and healthcare becomes no more than a place where sick people work on sick people.

And there is nothing to be proud of in that.

In order to be compassionate to others, first you must be compassionate to yourself.

That is the bottom line.

Burnout is no more than the complete demoralisation of the compassionate person.

There are no winners in that.

Just an ever-flowing ebb tide of suffering.

This book is about teaching clinicians compassionate systems of work, from a very unique perspective and a very unique starting point.

Below Ten Thousand is a profound gauge of workplace culture.

The less safe the culture, the less compassionate the culture, the less 'just' the culture, the less chance of 'bringing it in'.

In the event of resistance, all is not lost.

Nothing worthwhile is easy, and resistance on the part of our own governance team, for yet unspecified reasons, enlightened us to the path of clinician-led culture change.

You already have all the permission you need
to be the change you want to see in your workplace.

And so it is that John and I discovered that change is a personal journey, and that, if the organisation is the sum of its people, then the people themselves can make the decision to change for the better, most importantly for themselves, but also for the patients.

Rome wasn't built in one day,
but Pompeii was buried in one.

And so it arises that whilst culture change in the direction of a more compassionate system may seem impossible, it is only impossible if no one takes that brave first step of empowering themselves.

WHY CLINICIAN-LED CULTURE CHANGE?

Clinicians exist at the clinical interface of every healthcare organisation. They are the enablers of everything that gets done.

They are the people who patients, their loved ones and, indeed, entire stratified healthcare organisations, depend upon to enhance and validate their existence. There is no better guardian to wellbeing than a clinician. Impeccable performance, for us, is essential.

There is no room for mistakes, nor oversights, nor errors of judgement.

In a healthcare system heavy with the burden of care, nurses comprise less than half the workforce and shoulder a vastly disproportionate percentage of the frontline burden.

Workplace culture is something beyond the metrics of power. It cannot be 'ordered' to exist. It arises from people and how they behave.

Some administrators feel threatened when the clinicians they direct come up with new ideas.

Some take action via avoidance, but the worst take action via oppression to undermine the innovator and their initiative.

Derailment is sometimes as simple as a single manager or director saying 'this won't work', thus sparing themselves the effort of even trying.

And sadly many of us are so easily dissuaded from what

we know to be right that such a simple throw-away line is enough to scuttle our progress.

Ultimately, it is the clinicians themselves who become responsible for the propagation of a positive organisational culture. Heavily burdened and far removed from executive decision making, they sadly imagine themselves to be powerless.

However, clinicians already have all the permission they need to be the change they want to see in their workplace.

All that is left is to make the decision to act.

Clinicians are trained to advocate on behalf of their patients. Advocating on behalf of themselves is more difficult. However, advocating for yourself IS advocating for your patient.

Empowerment is the key, and clinician-led culture change is the key to the future.

'First do no harm' is a central tenet of our work. But when it comes to entering a hospital, harm is everywhere and occurs on a daily basis, not just to patients but to staff as well. There is room for improvement and that improvement must come from you.

Below Ten Thousand is a simple example of cultural improvement led by clinicians.

Patients of the future will not just want it, they will *demand* it of the teams enacting their care.

Clinician-led culture change will save lives. But first we must embrace the courage to change.

If evidence suggests Iatrogenic Misadventure may be the third highest cause of death, as it does, we can no longer afford to be ignorant, arrogant nor complacent.

CASE STUDY #1:
CATEGORY ONE CAESAREAN SECTION

Chaos.

A patient crashes through the door with two midwives in tow.

There is the delivery bed, the baby cot, the foetal heart monitor, the copious notes, the stunned birthing partner, the screaming mother-to-be.

The theatre techs are scurrying to get equipment.

At the same time some of the hurriedly-assembled team are moving the patient on to the theatre table whilst protecting the urinary catheter and the drip.

The surgical team prep and drape and get knife to skin but the paediatrician and paediatric registrar are talking in one corner, the midwives are joining in, the techs are comparing notes on Caesar Theatre setup for different surgeons, the anaesthetists are discussing whatever anaesthetists discuss and the scouts are calling through the open door for another bowl set.

The noise is so loud that Kathy, the scrub nurse, is having trouble hearing the surgeon.

She looks up, scans the room, takes in the situation. The baby is not yet out and tension fringed with frustration is evident on the surgeon's face.

Kathy takes a breath.

'Below Ten Thousand!'

The room immediately quiets.

Everyone in the room becomes 100% present to the task at hand.

The surgical team can focus, communicate and function better together and surgery goes from 'clunky' to 'flow'.

The baby is delivered and all proceeds uneventfully to the end of the case.

TWENTY-FIVE WORDS OR LESS

After our first presentation to the anaesthetists, John and I were in the corridor debriefing. Dean Dimovski, a cardiac anaesthetist, came running by.

Dean was breathless:

'I really wanted to hear your talk but I got caught up! I'm in a hurry but if you can give me your talk in 25 words or less, I'd like to hear it now!'

I looked at John and John looked at me.

John thinks better on his feet and is the better communicator, so I deferred to him. 'Be my guest.'

John said:

'Immediate, unquestioned quiet when you need it most.

All you have to do is ask.

The words to use are "Below Ten Thousand".'

Dean laughed. 'I want it!' he exclaimed. 'And ... you still have two words left.'

John thought about it for a moment.

'The End,' he concluded.

CASE STUDY #2:
FESTIVE CHEER

It's Christmas Day.

The surgical team are taking biopsies during a gastroscopy.

The proceduralist advances the biopsy forceps. 'Open ... close ...' He tugs on the wire, hoping to have snared a good tissue sample.

The rest of the staff in the room are cheerfully engaged in Christmas banter.

Anthea, the scrub nurse, is having trouble hearing the instructions.

'Hey, guys. Below Ten Thousand!'

Staff immediately comply.

Someone grumbles.

The anaesthetist support Anthea's call.

'She's right. Let's focus.'

A look of relief is evident on Anthea's face.

She didn't want to be a party pooper, but the distraction was making her job very difficult.

Later, a nurse apologises to Anthea for his part of the noise in the room.

Sometimes it's easy to forget where we are and we allow ourselves to get carried away. It's important to recognise and take ownership of our lapses when we do that.

BEST PRACTICE

According to Wikipedia:

A best practice is a method or technique that has consistently shown results superior to those achieved with other means, and that is used as a benchmark. In addition, a 'best' practice can evolve to become better as improvements are discovered.

Best practice is considered by some as a business buzzword, used to describe the process of developing and following a standard way of doing things that multiple organisations can use.

Best practices are used to maintain quality as an alternative to mandatory legislated standards and can be based on self-assessment or benchmarking. A key strategic talent required when applying best practice to organisations is the ability to balance the unique qualities of an organisation with the practices that it has in common with others.

BEST PRACTICE AND BELOW TEN THOUSAND

Below Ten Thousand fills a void in 'situational awareness team-focusing triggers' which are absent from operating theatres and, indeed, healthcare settings everywhere.

At its inception it was developed to address the unresolved issue of noise and distraction behaviours in the operating theatres.

It was one important step beyond that reached by all

professional thinking at the time. Articles were slowly appearing suggesting the introduction of the 'Sterile Cockpit' into operating theatre culture. The authors of these documents, however, were unable to visualise or create a 'working actualiser'.

We were able to envisage the concept and to engineer a way of making it work in the cultural construct of clinical practice.

At this point in time, with the dire need for new cultural directions in healthcare, Below Ten Thousand places clinicians who adopt the initiative in a global leadership role with respect to operating theatre safety and quality practices.

Rob Tomlinson, a Junior Nurse Manager at the Royal Blackburn Hospital in the United Kingdom found himself in such a position when he decided to implement it at his hospital. The clinical safety leadership role was an unanticipated consequence.

Rob soon found himself in demand, initially throughout the East Lancashire Health Trust and then right across the NHS as other hospitals became aware of his documented success at significantly reducing errors and harm in patients in his hospital.

Incidental support was provided by a change in NHS strategic direction.

The NHS realised that a substantial barrier to patient safety was the glass wall inadvertently constructed by the significant hierarchical levels that exist within patient care teams. This cultural barrier prevented junior staff from speaking up when they saw something that might compromise patient safety.

The barrier creates errors of omission and errors of commission that serve to jeopardise good patient outcomes and demonstrably results in iatrogenic patient harm.

Below Ten Thousand effectively serves to:

- flatten the hierarchy
- de-escalate the emotion
- give a safe voice to each person in the room, and
- evokes a behavioural response that accords with best practice.

It provided the cultural change the NHS needed.

It was free, validated and so, so easy for the conscientious clinician to at once both apply and comply.

If adopted in full, it had the potential to prevent iatrogenic complications as well as reduce high cost litigation. If payouts of £45 million pounds could be prevented for free, you'd want it too!

Cultural best practice is more than free.

It saves lives and careers as well as money.

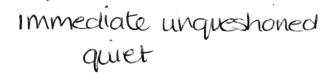

Immediate unquestioned
quiet

THE UNDERBELLY OF THEATRES

Anna was a talented, passionate, nursing student. She was always going to make an amazing perioperative nurse.

Now qualified and working in the operating theatre, Anna continues to be a great nurse.

She loves her work. She loves her colleagues. She loves the idea of surgically fixing people.

Despite these loves, Anna unscrubbed from an operation the other day in tears because of conflict going on between people in the room.

It is so sad because both Anna and her patient deserve so much better.

In my opinion, if I were that patient and if I had a poor outcome from that operation I'd sue the bullies *and* the organisation.

An organisational culture that allows such negative behaviour to occur is negligent in three ways:

1. It is negligent in the provision of an effective safety culture which ensures delivery of safe care for the patient

2. It is negligent in the provision of a safe workplace for Anna

3. And if conflict is demonstrably pervasive, it is negligent in the governance of those duties of care.

THE 'REASONABLE PERSON' TEST

In making judgements when adjudicating negligence in the clinical setting, the decision is based around the 'reasonable person' test.

In simple terms, the reasonable person test seeks to determine what the average nurse would do in such a situation.

Not the worst.

Not the best.

But what the 'reasonable person' would do.

If the reasonable person would behave in a way that seeks to minimise diversions from process and distractions from the task at hand, then so be it.

If the reasonable person can argue:

I have the right to tolerate breakdown and disregard noise and distraction as a critical element of the safety environment.

then maybe we are not as clever as we think we are.

PRINCIPLES OF
BELOW TEN THOUSAND

The term 'Below Ten Thousand' is borrowed from the 'Sterile Cockpit' and refers in an aeronautical context to the time a plane is between the ground and an altitude of ten thousand feet.

Think of a plane skimming the tree tops.

This is the time during which focus on the task at hand and prevention of distractions is most critical.

The successful navigation of complex time-critical and vital task sets requires a high degree of competence executed within a setting of high pressure and high cognitive load.

The phrase 'Below Ten Thousand' is a trigger phrase, a generic 'safe word' that can be used by anyone.

It precipitates an effective behavioural response in all members of the team when voiced to the room.

It simply requests a reduction in non-essential conversation, complete focus on the task at hand and increased situational awareness at key and pivotal times.

It was originally developed for use by anaesthetic teams at induction and extubation, but quickly evolved to include scrub counts, the World Health Organisation (WHO) Surgical Safety Checklist, and any time 'a moment to think' is required.

Dr Carol-Anne Moulton's work on 'slowing down moments' features strongly.

In the operating theatre, 'Below Ten Thousand' is used as a non-confrontational and non-conflictive verbal tool to effect behavioural team competence at those times when ambient noise and distraction erode the safety and reliability of clinical team performance.

It serves to optimise effective team behaviours in a multidisciplinary team comprising individuals with offset periods of activity and inactivity.

At its core are the dual ethical paradigms of advocacy and trust.

Put simply, 'Below Ten Thousand' creates a safe working environment by reducing ambient noise and refocusing the team.

It has the potential to immediately reduce non-task related distractions, making concentration and communication more effective and less effortful.

It bears a 'Stop, Look and Listen' motif which also serves as an early-escalation graded assertiveness tool.

And it asks the question of each and every team member:

'How do you choose to function within and as a team?'

The behavioural answer to that question is not always consistent with an individual's self-ascribed beliefs and values.

This final realisation is why cultural evolution in our clinical environment is so important.

It redirects our thinking from an illusion which we believe to be true to a concrete construct that in reality *is* true.

CASE STUDY #3:
HAPPILY VALIDATED

Carol is an anaesthetist.

She is also a vocal supporter of her local football team. At the footy she has no trouble finding her voice and she can yell and scream with the best of them.

In the operating theatre she tends to be more reserved. Quiet.

Being young and female she realises that it can be difficult to tread that fine line between being 'nice' (read 'gently assertive') and being considered 'a bitch' when trying to exert authority in the pressure-cooker environment of the operating room.

In the past, when she tried to quiet a room full of busy people before putting an anxious patient off to sleep, she would generally fail.

She would carry on the induction in substandard conditions, feeling flustered, which is sad because she values highly her ability to talk calmly and reassuringly to her patients, to 'whisper them off to sleep', so to speak.

Later in the day of the Below Ten Thousand inservice she calls 'Below Ten Thousand' in the theatre.

Later, her smile proclaims her happiness. 'It worked!' she exclaims to her assistant.

She felt heard, validated and supported in her desire to provide exceptional care for her patient.

CLINICIAN-LED CULTURE CHANGE

A WORTHWHILE CHALLENGE

It doesn't matter how junior you are and it doesn't matter how skilful you are, because we are all human and no one person is more human than any other.

Despite our desire for empathy, we don't often consider the limits of our own humanity.

In the heroic model of healthcare, we all expect to be superhuman.

But as any exercise physiologist will tell you, the human body has limitations.

As any cognitive psychologist will tell you, the human mind has limitations.

And as any Below Ten Thousand practitioner will tell you, the more we push the limits of our cognitive and physiological capacities, the more we approach the event horizon which is the 'edge of coping', beyond which there is clinician suffering.

Compassion is the ability to empathise with another's suffering. Therefore, a compassionate system must be able to take into consideration its participants' suffering and engineer systems architectures which prevent, as much as possible, that suffering.

Systems sustainability can be mapped mathematically.

Inputs and outputs can be quantified and verified.

The mathematics needed to arrive at the answer is easy.

Working out what should be *in* the equation?

Now *that's* the difficult part.

Clinician-led culture change is about filling in the gaps of those equations.

It is about giving a voice to those working at the clinical interface who identify an opportunity to improve the way we do the things we do.

It is a much more personal journey than we may have thought and is centred around how each of us behaves within our system of work, and how we perform our body of knowledge.

Whilst traditionally we have centred our work around processes that have evolved as a legacy of archaic solutions to historical problems, modern clinical environments are now so empirically different.

The exponential escalation of technology and the increasing complexity of procedural interventions means that our systems of work and human factors thinking have been severely outpaced by the current period of intense transition we are living through.

The thing that has to change is our thinking.

And the thing that has to change about our thinking is that, whilst technology and learning remain the dominant progressive forces in our clinical lives, our humanity remains the same.

Therefore, organisational thinking has to take into account this simple matter:

'How do we mould our processes around our people in order to keep our people safe and effective in everything they do?'

And our personal thinking has to take into account this simple matter:

'How do I mould my behaviour in order to keep *me* safe and effective in everything I do?'

Because whilst doing compulsory annual competency testing and professional education may permit you to continue to practice, these things won't keep you from crying at the end of each day.

THE HALF-LIFE OF MEDICAL KNOWLEDGE

The half-life of medical knowledge is anecdotally seven years.

It has been suggested that in seven years, half of what you thought you knew is obsolete, superseded or just plain wrong.

The rate of advance in medical practice and the technology associated with it is incredible and with it, the challenge to stay current is huge.

When John and I introduced the idea of Below Ten Thousand to our colleagues, we understood we were competing for cognitive bandwidth in a *very* congested marketplace.

We knew we had about thirty seconds to engage our colleagues before their attention moved on to the next thing on their busy agenda.

The image of a plane skimming the treetops was a very powerful one and we hoped it would lodge a memorable cognitive association deep within their minds.

COLLABORATION

HIGH PERFORMANCE TEAMS?

The endpoint of Below Ten Thousand is the construction of high performance teams.

But steady on!

The thing to be careful about here is that we often have an image in mind when talking in terms of a strong sporting metaphor. We think that in order to construct a high performance team we need only stack the team with champions.

But we want something much more realistic and robust than that.

For us, a high performance team is a team of ordinary people who function well together in a system of work where processes are simple and flow; and in which obstacles to flow and redundant complexities have been eliminated.

A high performance team has a tangible 'best practice' outcome in mind and the whole entity behaves in such a way that it reliably reinforces that outcome.

A high performance team doesn't hide its mistakes, it learns from them. It understands that barriers to open communication are dangerous. Therefore, in the absence of malicious negligence, there is no blame.

High performance team environments can only be so if the participants are honest, exemplify trust, and are in optimal performance condition.

With respect to individual performance:

The body works best when it is fed, watered, given

opportunities to rest and timely opportunities for elimination (loo breaks).

The brain works best when it is fed, watered, given opportunities to rest and timely opportunities for offloading (debriefing).

Looking after staff in these matters allows them to function better.

Bringing the responsibility home, looking after yourself in these matters, allows you to function better.

Being able to operate within the limits of sustainability ensures you have adequate energy to function well at work.

Being able to operate within the limits of sustainability ensures you have adequate energy to function well at home.

Both home and work sustain each other. There is no dichotomy. Dysfunction in either life brings suffering.

Being able to operate within the limits of sustainability ensures you have adequate energy to function well in all aspects of your life.

A HOSED DOWN HIERARCHY

Clinical nurses, traditionally, are right down there at the bottom of the pecking order. Empirically we get the worst hours, the worst car parks, the worst workloads, the worst blame.

Clinical nursing is 'the beat' and from there, promotion is the only thing that will lift us out of the mind and body-numbing fatigue of 'getting things done' on a 24/7 circadian-toxic rotating roster.

The higher up the chain of command you go, the more decisions you get to make about what nurses do and how they do it.

Except that from the glass walls of power, memory fades.

The only remnant left after a while is the subconscious demand that 'you never want to go back there again'.

In terms of positional power, clinical nurses exert little.

Power is dissipated by the ethical code of our unspoken social contract, reflected in the nursing oath that each takes upon graduation.

In terms of 'getting things done', however, nurses are right at the top of the chart.

So arise some interesting thoughts:

'Why do we disempower the very people entrusted with doing the work?'

'Why do we afford them so little creativity when they know intimately what gets in the way of them doing their job?'

Instead, we fit the person around the work instead of fitting the work around what is humanly reasonable.

There is a tale about a frog in a pot of water.

It is possible for the frog to leave at any time.

Heat up the water and the frog remains.

By the time the water becomes scalding, the frog can no longer escape and thus boils to death.

There are a number of worthy discussion points in this parable.

1. Whoever does this experiment lacks compassion for frogs.
2. Frogs become tolerant of increasingly toxic conditions.
3. Frogs die if they don't make a decision to save themselves before the damage becomes irreversible.

Student nurses become immersed in our clinical culture. All they want to do is fit in.

By the time they have enough experience to take action, they are so inoculated to the way things are that they assume that is the way things have to be.

They may not get boiled alive, but they may get 'eaten alive' by their colleagues or burned out by the weight of expectation.

I've often heard the saying that 'Nurses eat their young'. Maybe this is what the saying means.

In the hierarchy of 'doing things' nurses are right at the top of the chain. All we have to do is teach nurses human factors and ergonomics and give them a voice that reimagines the future.

This is the essence of clinician-led culture change.

It's not that hard.

Managers need not worry.

Managers are not out of a job. In fact, they will be working more effectively than ever.

As the saying goes, managers are communicated *through*, not communicated *to*!

Middle managers now get to advocate up the chain of command as well as down, rather than the traditional one-way flow of issuing commands.

All they need is courage, wisdom, imagination and passion.

Supporting a clinician-led initiative brings great opportunities and coaching a team brings great rewards.

Part of the reward is derived from seeing people function at their best.

And although it may seem frightening to let nurses create input into systems of work that facilitate getting the job done, managers don't have to worry.

Nurses are not interested in breaking the system.

They are only interested in doing their best.

The nursing oath takes care of that.

ENGAGEMENT

The introduction of any clinician-led culture change is best served by a number of educational strategies.

The most important realisation for John and I was that we were competing in a congested marketplace for cognitive bandwidth. Our approach had to be tailored to that effect.

We needed to capture attention and deliver memorable content in thirty seconds, which is all busy people would give us unless we arrested their intrigue sufficiently to make them stop and engage.

Guerrilla marketing strategies became our friend as we marketed in-house to our peers.

Engagement in a clinician-led project is all about good faith, because that is the only collateral we have to work with.

And since nursing is a human science and we are seeking to influence human behaviour to the positive, the principles of Game Theory come in to play.

Game Theory mathematically depicts behaviour between two self-interested parties, where each party gets to choose their own level of engagement for their own anticipated payoffs.

There will always be early adopters, late adopters and those who will actively resist all attempts to persuade. Knowing this makes it easier to develop your networking and educational strategies. You just need to build a growing tide of change to help dilute resistance.

RELATIONSHIP BUILDING

Informal conversation with like-minded peers is a great way to sow the seeds of change.

Conversation allows you to find like-minded souls and early adopters because culture change needs friends.

A groundswell of interest is a great springboard from which to launch your campaign to introduce the Below Ten Thousand Way. It is easier, then, to approach your managers because you have a fully formed plan:

You know the need exists.

You know the interest is there.

You have all the materials you need at hand.

And – you have a plan.

Finally, it helps if your manager needs a rubber-stamped fully-fledged quality and safety improvement project to undertake to help them satisfy accreditation requirements, and it helps if that plan arrives in their office with ready-made content and a fully informed project leader.

That's *you*!

Fair warning: as simple as Below Ten Thousand is, there is a lot of work involved that simply gets layered over the top of normal clinical workloads.

Ashley Kirk from Dunedin got around this problem by forming a steering committee to drive the change. Smart guy, that Ash.

FORMAL PRESENTATIONS

Presentations on Below Ten Thousand should be delivered initially by the project leaders and should include all operating theatre staff, either separately or as a group.

They should be given to nurses, technicians, surgeons, anaesthetists and out-of-department visitors to the theatre suite (e.g. midwives, paediatricians, radiographers).

SIGNAGE

Posters and visual signage are available for free from the www.belowtenthousand.com website, although it is much more solid fun should you wish to create your own.

The greatest way of clinician-led team building is to invite colleagues with artistic abilities to help – and embrace their talents.

The excitement and conversation that surrounds such creative collaboration has much intrinsic value. This type of engagement is far more effective at breaking the ice than any amount of ordinary educational 'pleading'.

PAMPHLETS

Tri-fold pamphlets created to quickly orientate new staff to the meaning and practice of Below Ten Thousand are also available and free to download from the website.

ORIENTATION

All new staff members including doctors commencing work in the operating theatre should have Below Ten Thousand training as a critical component of their orientation program.

This should be delivered by the educator or orientation facilitator and be on the checklist of competencies to be delivered.

MEASUREMENT

Our data collection instrument was by survey.

Our survey was simple.

It took 1 minute and 4 seconds to complete.

It measured any perceived improvement in the safety environment, as well as the circumstances of use.

The one thing we didn't want to do was burden people with more paperwork.

And since Below Ten Thousand was a voluntary 'opt in' project, we were reliant upon goodwill and the momentum of enthusiasm amid all the other pressures of clinical practice in order to collect our data.

Therefore, we had to be happy with n=10 on our first attempt, which made it no more than a pilot study.

Rob Tomlinson at East Lancashire Hospital Trust did much, much better.

His n=50 study produced affirming data, showing marked improvement to safe patient care delivery.

Whilst, more formal research is needed to validate our findings that Below Ten Thousand provides a working environment that is more conducive to safer patient management, Rob Tomlinson, in collaboration with the AfPP, is currently working towards establishing a firmer evidentiary base.

Whatever their findings, their collaboration will create strong foundations for a safer future.

ON-SELLING

Sometimes you have to sell a concept to the world in order to sell it to your own colleagues.

Others benefit from learning your story and witnessing the improvements to team culture and safety you have made.

Your colleagues get to develop a sense of pride in having their achievements recognised.

Celebrate your success by presenting a poster or a talk at a conference, or by writing about your experience in professional journals.

Such acts further best practice.

Such efforts showcase your character strengths.

Such efforts serve to construct a portfolio of your professional abilities, aptitudes and values.

'Share and the world shares with you,' they say!

FURTHER POTENTIAL

Once the Below Ten Thousand team behaviour strategy is in place and is being effectively utilised, more advanced team behaviour improvement strategies may then be explored.

Below Ten Thousand is the first step on the path toward the creation of the high performance team, since it gets everyone to start thinking about how each and every individual performs within and as a team.

Just when you think you are done, you realise you are just getting started.

No matter. Re-energise yourself and celebrate your wins along the way.

In fifty years' time I would hope that historians will be horrified by the injustices that occurred at that time in that hospital which stood like an edifice of death overlooking a regional city of parochial ordinariness.

Conflict is a failure of logic.

I had a dream last night. In it, centurions fought their last remaining rebels, brutally overcoming them and in doing so attaining the endgame of peace through total subjugation.

And amid the tangle of broken bodies and spears, a soldier realised the ignorant dystopian intractability of the massacre with the lament: 'What have we done??!!!'

What we have done in healthcare is simple.

It takes a world of people to make a hospital. It takes a world of ordinary people doing exceptional things. And instead of helping those people to their feet we have kept them on their knees on broken glass.

We have set up a colony no better than that in 'Lord of the Flies', when so much better has been, was, and always is, possible.

Was Dante correct when he said, 'Abandon hope, all ye who enter here.'?

And was it a warning or just good advice?

I take my heart from Milton.

> *The mind is its own place, and in itself,*
> *can make a Heaven of Hell, a Hell of Heaven.*
> *What matter where, if I be still the same?*

Who cares where?
I care.

ROGUES OF SAFETY

John and I developed and marketed the Below Ten Thousand concept to our colleagues at the hospital where we worked and it was enthusiastically received.

From there it has spread worldwide thanks to the Herculean efforts of wonderful people. But it wasn't always a smooth ride.

We tried to include our managers at every step of our concept development, but they refused to engage, and as we progressed they became resentful of our work.

It's not unusual for new ideas to meet a hostile reception in their formative location, but we were surprised to be labelled 'rogues' by our own leadership team when we did so much to try to include them from the very outset, as per our ethic of open collaboration.

In the end, despite 90 percent of the clinical staff being educated in the concept, enthusiastically using the tool and clamouring for its official stamp of approval from the bosses, that stamp of approval never eventuated. And with our educator too scared to promote it at orientation, perpetuation of the tool to successive generations of new staff became problematic.

John and I were told emphatically, 'All you have is three words and when you leave they will die.'

But we continued to push our cause because we considered it unethical not to. Patients (and staff) were still being compromised by noise and distraction, and even though we continued to invest time, energy and money into keeping the clinician-led cultural change at the forefront of clinicians' working knowledge, we figured that hospital would never be a primary 'customer'.

We had our first big break when Liverpool Hospital in Sydney gave us an overwhelming thumbs up and their Director of Nursing labelled Below Ten Thousand 'a very patient-centric Model of Care'.

Our second big break came from the Pennsylvania Patient Safety Authority acknowledging our work, and this was complemented soon after by the arrival on the scene of Rob Tomlinson from the UK and Ash Kirk from New Zealand.

Rob's advocacy got a boost, first from the AfPP who labelled Below Ten Thousand 'the missing link in the Surgical Safety Checklist' and more recently from the Care Quality Commission who included it as a safety strategy in their 2019 'Prevention of Never Events' report.

Ash's outcome was awesome, too.

At Dunedin Mercy, Below Ten Thousand was approved for use right throughout the hospital in clinical and non-clinical settings and has the vocal backing of the CEO.

John and I knew we would have to sell the concept to the world in order to sell it to our own operating theatre management team, and that's what we still vow to do.

To illustrate our lack of progress at our own institution, I heard that a year ago a junior nurse in the day surgery unit spoke at a meeting about something she had read in the 'Journal of Perioperative Nursing', and how she thought it would be a great idea to introduce it into her work setting.

She was puzzled by the complete lack of enthusiasm for her request from her operating services manager and educator, and it was only later that the nurse learned that the project she was talking about, Below Ten Thousand, had its birthplace 150 metres away and three floors up in the main operating theatre of her own hospital.

Likewise, when Rob's award win was mentioned by a nurse at a general theatre staff meeting, the clinical staff went wild with applause.

The management team, however, remained mute.

One of the reasons I left was because of the strain of the oppositional management culture and their relentless hostility towards clinicians.

I felt I could no longer effectively advocate for my friends (conflict resolution) and patients (safety). I could no longer function in that deeply absurd environment and it is only two and a half years later that I feel 'healed' in some way and now only rarely dream about it.

I hope my story doesn't diminish the reader's respect for that carefully deliberated idea that John Gibbs innovated and that I, naturally, plunged headlong into making a reality irrespective of the consequences.

Some might say I am an idiot.

Some might say I was brave.

But in the end, ethics is simply a call to do the right thing, and the cost means nothing when what is at stake is a matter of heart.

I'm not ashamed to have been branded a 'Rogue of Safety'.

PLAN; DO; CHECK; BUILD

John and I made up a 'High Performance Team Wheel'.

It formed the basis of our Below Ten Thousand modus operandi for introducing change into the clinical setting, and through it we sought to encourage innovators to involve and empower other clinicians in the finding of lasting solutions to 'systems of work' problems.

The wheel takes us from 'idea' to 'goal' in an inclusive and cooperative way, engineering trust and collaboration into the change process.

Through feedback we were able to evaluate the outcome achieved by our innovation and use our accumulated learning to facilitate our next improvement effort.

The light hand of management is merely to facilitate the process, to touch but not stamp on the process.

Because you can't brute force effective change.

PHASE 1

From the generation of an idea, the High Performance Team Wheel takes us through the magic question:

'So, what would such a thing *look like*?'

This phase, Phase 1, is the birthing phase.

Or perhaps it's the Demise Phase if an idea proves untenable.

The task of reverse engineering the process uses the contextual experience of those actually *doing* the work.

Individuals who work every day at the clinical interface know the true limiting and enhancing factors: the rules, regulations and behaviours that serve to optimise or break the flow of their work.

Frontline workers must firstly give themselves the authority to critique their own practices and that of their peers, and secondly they must *give a damn*!!!

They have to *want* to be the vehicles of the change *they* want to see, not just wander around and believe that *management* will make or change rules for the better.

The goal is the creation of humanistic and sustainable decision-making trees which are mindful of outcome.

Success depends on the presence or creation of trust and the willingness to invest in the workplace and those who work within it.

This is *engagement*, just in case we need to spell out what engagement really means.

There is one more important distinction:

Engagement must be 'in fact, not just 'in appearance'!

And listening is often the hardest skill to master.

Once you have a handle on the proposed process, the next phase, Phase 2, is to build collaboration and thus ownership of the solution.

PHASE 2

Here we build the solution to its most architecturally sound and effective form.

In terms of Below Ten Thousand, we started off with the aim of having 'immediate, unquestioned quiet'.

Through collaboration we matured that aim.

We found out that what was required was the immediate creation of a problem solving environment.

This included not just 'noise and distraction abatement', but the refocusing of situational awareness and the manifesting of a high performance team environment which sometimes involved cross-disciplinary communication coupled with exchange of ideas and information.

Same general idea, but with a stronger, more strategic and empowering purpose and outcome.

Note that buy-in from other people also increases ownership of the idea as it creates discussion and essentially coaches collaboration.

The process allows systems learning because, having done it once, we can use the trust engineered to solve problems in a better way, more easily, more resolutely and faster the next time around.

The 'fear' barrier to change has been broken, since change mechanics at the clinical level now includes participation and terms of reference, not just imposition.

We incorporated into Phase 2 the cycle of:

- Plan your strategy
- Do what you say you will
- Check that it works
- Build on the collaborative feedback.

At each cycle, you build on what you had before and check that it works. The skill in this building process is the understanding of what we call 'uncompl3xity', or the engineering of elegance into the process.

You know when you are finished, not when there is nothing left to add, but when there is nothing left to take away.

The final result is fluid, doable, effective, efficient, solid, and maximally responsive to downstream systems flow.

There is no futility.

The Below Ten Thousand definition of futility?

'Process dismissive of outcome!'

You will know what I mean when you see it.

CASE STUDY #6:
INTENSIVE CARE

The nurses in Intensive Care found out about Below Ten Thousand.

A group of likeminded individuals discussed the possibilities.

'You know, the biggest problem I have every day is when the cardiac surgery patient arrives. Everyone is so busy getting things organised that no one gets to hear the whole story, then everyone disappears and I'm like, 'What just happened?'

The nurses took their discussion to the intensive care doctors, who agreed.

'Let's just make the whole transition of care event a Below Ten Thousand moment,' they concurred.

So instead of a flurry of activity when the next patient arrived, everyone listened and observed the patient until handover was complete.

Then the team got on with their jobs with everyone equally clear about the ongoing expectations for the patient's care.

'That's just blown me away,' one nurse remarked.

'For the first time I just saw the patient as a person rather than as a series of jobs to do.

'Right now, I feel even more proud to be part of the team I'm in!'

PHASE 3

Now that we have the finished product, replete with inbuilt ownership established through collaboration, we move into the next phase which is incorporation of the idea into practice and its perpetuation into culture.

This is the 'building capacity in your team' part.

We now know the idea will never stall because ownership ensures that it will be passed on to each new wave of clinicians as they pass through on their clinical journey.

In this, we have achieved our goal and created dynamic team resilience, because if they can solve one problem, they can solve another.

Arriving at a goal demands celebration.

Not of you, silly, but of *them*!

They created the change and achieved the goal!

It might seem the long way around, but it is a *sustainable* result.

It seems like a helluva long way 'round!

The temptation is to take the short cut, to go the wrong way around the wheel, straight from 'idea' to 'goal' without all the clinician input. From a manager's perspective, that temptation is *strong*.

Less effort coupled with maximum delegation.

It feels so right.

But that is building 'command and control', which is not as good as building 'trust'.

And building a body of 'Because I said so' responses is not as effective as building a body of 'empowerment mindful of the ultimate shared goal' ones.

This is all scary stuff, because it flies in the face of our understanding of the idea of 'being a strong leader'.

But if high performance teams of clinicians are sustainably solving clinical flow dilemmas, then each solution becomes one less 'fire' you will have to put out tomorrow, which frees up more time to manage and lead and develop better contingency strategies, identify and grow talent and plan for the future.

It is, in the end, building process, culture and authenticity from the ground up, which is a damn sight better than distrust, disengagement, hypocrisy, disconnect and chaos.

To move forward to a more mature and strategic future, first you must be intellectually humble.

Then you can wisely lead your team of empowered systems engineers into a brave new world.

CASE STUDY #7:
'IF IT ONLY SAVES YOU ONCE A YEAR'

A surgeon is operating and blood loss is becoming a concern.

Everyone is busy concentrating on other things, and no one seems to be paying attention to his request for blood.

He is getting frustrated and is on the point of exploding.

Instead, he takes a deep breath.

'Below Ten Thousand!' he calls.

A discussion occurs. Blood is fetched, the transfusions are commenced and the resuscitation efforts continue.

Surgery is successfully completed due to the dexterity and skill of the surgical team.

As the surgeon flicks his gloves into the bin, he confides in his registrar:

'I never thought I would use it, but calling "Below Ten Thousand" has saved me a trip to HR. Thank God, because I've got a million other things to do and I don't need the distraction of dealing with them.

'I guess if it only saves me once a year, it's a good year!'

'WITHIN AND AS A TEAM'

I was mentoring an undergraduate nursing student in Recovery one day. I asked her what work she had done prior to embarking on her nursing career.

She apologised for the fact that she had only been a housemaid at a local resort town hotel.

'There is no need to apologise,' I replied. 'Tell me about your job.'

The more she told me, the more I was able to reflect back to her character strengths that made her a good team player who had an eye for envisioning and enacting high quality outcomes.

She seemed surprised but happy with our conversation, and by the end of the day her confidence in engaging with patients in the scary environment of the Post Anaesthesia Care Unit was vastly improved.

Improved confidence meant she learned better, she observed better, she engaged better, and she responded to changing circumstances in ways that were proactive and measured rather than panicked.

All we had done was reflect on her ability to perform within and as part of a team.

It was that reassurance that led her to become an excellent nurse.

I met Gabby again many years later in an operating theatre 1650 kilometres away.

Gabby reflected on her learning:

'I still recall the award you gave me when I successfully

managed my first obstructed airway. You made me wear that sticker all day, and everybody commented on it.'

It was a simple gesture, but the message was delivered:

'Anchor yourself in time and place; and learn and act confidently within your advancing knowledge and skill sets.

'And celebrate your achievements, no matter how small.

'Trust adds another strand to the string that secures the Damocles sword.'

Gabby got stronger, felt safer, felt part of a team, and so became less fearful and more resilient.

It is *through* people like Gabby that we worked out our vision for the Below Ten Thousand Way.

It is *with thanks to* people like Gabby that we can write this book.

It is *for people* like Gabby that we demand a better way, because we want people like Gabby to be the best they can be.

Not just the best the system's culture allows her to be.

Working within a flawless team is an ambition to which we as operating theatre nurses subscribe.

Flawless teams, however, take a lot of work and maintenance, which is difficult in an environment of overwhelming production pressure with legacy-riddled systems of work.

Instead, we spend a lot of energy each day overcoming obstacles and conflicts we inevitably put in our own way.

Smarter?

Safer?

Better?

I think we can do it, if only for people like Gabby.

FLAWLESS TEAMS

Leadership is, unfortunately, not always inspiring, supportive and inclusive.

In organisations with endemic cultural problems, the rot (or at least the fixed mindset arising from pretentious egoistic constructs), sets in from the top.

In recruitment, like tends to select like, and it only takes one sociopath to start the process of eroding the effectiveness of a whole department or even the entire organisation over time.

The best place to start when leadership fails you is with your Professional Standards.

Professional associations such as The Australian College of Operating Room Nurses (ACORN) spend a huge amount of effort constructing peer reviewed, evidence based standards for practice. These standards are comprehensive, considered and evolving. Fortunately, the standards are not only organisational guides for practice, they are personal guides for practice as well.

Despite executive focus on production pressure at the expense of all else, the standards keep you safe. Or at least they give you the evidence you need to ensure your practice remains safe.

Flawless teams do not arise from sociopathy. They arise from 'Just' cultures.

They arise from ordinary people who feel safe to function without the distraction of fear from irrational antisocial behaviours.

Put another way, they arise from ordinary people who feel secure to function proactively and with emotional intelligence within a rational system of work.

The difference is simply a matter of trust.

TRUST

Trust is the most basic common factor in flawless teams. Trust can be achieved with:

- effective compliance with Standards
- effective boundaries
- effective communication chains
- effective line management
- effective processes
- effective follow up
- effective review processes
- effective checking in to make sure everything is ok
- effective people.

If you are thinking that is too simple an explanation, don't worry.

If it was easy, everyone would be doing it.

BULLYING AS A DISTRACTION

Bullying is endemic in high risk, high pressure environments such as healthcare.

We never really think about bullying as a cognitive distraction from the task at hand.

But having to watch your back with every move, trying to concentrate despite the anxiety of hypercriticism, trying to think from within the fog of uncertainty created by illogical outbursts ...

All these things are distractions which erode your confidence and ability to work to a high performance level.

Thus bullying is unsafe, unwanted and unwarranted.

Bullying is as much a Below Ten Thousand moment as anything else.

CASE STUDY #8:
BEHIND THE BLOOD-BRAIN BARRIER

There is often a drape screen separating the surgical field from the anaesthetic field. This helps maintain the sterile surgical field.

Because the anaesthetist is often seated behind this 'curtain' (which came to be known as the 'blood-brain barrier'), they aren't always privy to the finer details of what is going on with the surgery, especially if there's a lot of noise and distraction.

At the end of one particularly noisy case, Ben, the surgeon, placed his gloves in the bin.

'Man, what a difficult case!'

Irena, the anaesthetist, looked at him quizzically.

'How so?' she asked.

'We were frantically dealing with a lot of generalised ooze.'

'Why didn't you call on "Below Ten Thousand"?' she asked. 'There are things I could have done that could have helped you with that, had I known.'

WORK FLOW
AND
INTENSIFICATION

CREATING FLOWING WORK DESIGNS

NEXT STEP THINKING AND UNC0MPL3XITY THEORY

Our tendency as humans is to overcomplicate things.

Over-complication often occurs to such a degree that it results in a disconnection between managers and workers.

This phenomenon occurs across all industries because neither protagonist believes the other has the ability to understand the complexities particular to their own work environment.

Despite our 'Lean' pretensions, we fail to enact the most simple rule of good design:

Perfect design occurs
not when there is nothing left to add,
but when there is nothing left to take away.

Healthcare is no different to any other industry in terms of efficiencies that may be gained from engineering simplicity into its systems and processes.

However, the extreme complexity of healthcare organisations conspires against the easy finding of simple solutions.

Nurses can be too caught up in the pedagogy to be able to permit themselves to offer useful solutions based upon their experiential insights.

Nurses, managers and clinicians alike are busy, boundary-constrained and indoctrinated people with many layers of complexity built into the work that they do.

They are trained to follow quite rigid and narrow sets of instructions and rules and trained to perform within specific narrow parameters of what constitutes 'safe' practice.

This is our default mode.

It constitutes our 'safe place'.

Because of these constraints, we don't think too much about how we do what we do.

Divergent thinking, even for the purposes of seeking improved clinical outcomes, traditionally comes at a heavy price.

We don't do advocacy well.

'Just do your work as you are trained to do it. Leave the thinking to others.'

As an example of 'others', it took a bricklayer to point out to operating theatre nurses how to better assist in an operation. If you don't believe me, just ask the bricklayer, Frank Bunker Gilbreth.

Further, we are convinced that complexity is good.

We have inherently found that intelligence built upon past intelligence creates a scenario where precedence informs future practice, and thus the smarter we get the more layers we apply and the more complex things become.

So this should deliver us better results.

Right?

Wrong.

What starts out looking good finishes up like a house made of cards – multilayered, impressive to look at, but functionally unstable.

At some point in time we need to deconstruct the historical edifice and reconstruct our work processes from a fresh design perspective.

As an example, let us look at a sandwich.

A sandwich is made from bread, which is basically a matrix of air and flour.

Bread is the saviour of civilisations.

A diet of bread and dripping got many people through periods of severe austerity.

It is so impressive, we even have a saying:

'The best thing since sliced bread.'

So bread is good. Right?

Better than bread is a salad sandwich.

Bread, lettuce, some grated carrot and tomato, a bit of beetroot and even a slice of ham.

Yum.

The salad sandwich was once the health food of a nation. Then came the next step.

No-one could agree on what should be in a salad sandwich.

White or multigrain?

Margarine or butter?

What sort of dressing?

Salt and pepper?

At least one mono-unsaturated fatty acid?

Ditch the ham?

Ditch the bread?

So on top of the original complexity came more complexity.

It became so complex that we no longer knew what was best.

Worse, I now may no longer care what I have for lunch.

It's all become too hard, so now I have a meat pie instead.

Healthcare is a bit like a salad sandwich.

Everything over time has become so complex and so busy that there is no time for variance and no tolerance for change.

Worse, pedagogy creates a culture of blame.

Now it is purported that half a nurse's time is spend dealing with the complexities of the system rather than dealing with the patient.

No wonder they are exhausted and frustrated and find it harder ... to ... care.

Into this realm strides Below Ten Thousand.

A short conversation about our desire to introduce into our operating theatre processes a simple entity called an intubation trolley delivers some conceptual rhetoric.

The idea of the trolley is not new and is so simple and basic to anaesthetic nursing that it is laughable.

What is even more laughable? John and I couldn't convince our managers to give us one.

The conceptual rhetoric, however, has powerful implications.

We started talking about how we go about the task of

intubating a patient, the distribution of our instruments, where they finish up, what else gets contaminated in the process and how that compromises our safety outcomes.

Then we came up with a framework:

Our framework was that our system of delivering an anaesthetic has three elements:

1. an intubating element
2. a gas delivery element, and
3. a drug delivery element.

The trouble we have is compounded by the fact that we don't separate out the elements.

We confuse them by bundling things all together in places they have no right to be, which makes following something as simple as a 'can't intubate, can't ventilate' algorithm superbly difficult.

Further, we reasoned, every workstation should tell its own story in its entirety, and *only* its own story in its entirety.

We came to the conclusion that to sort out our mess, and in fact to sort out any mess that any anaesthetic simulator or, dare I say it, any real life scenario could throw at us at any given time and without any given warning, we needed every workstation to have one purpose, and to be fully prepared for that one purpose.

In anaesthetics, there is only one cold, hard fact:

Any patient is ever only three minutes from death.

As a next step, we took the anaesthetic drug trolley and conceptually reconstructed the ampoule layout so that the drugs needed at the start of an anaesthetic were on the left hand side of the drawer, the drugs needed for the middle of the anaesthetic were in the middle of the drawer, and the drugs needed at the end of the case were on the right hand side of the drawer.

And so the drawer told the narrative of the case as we progressed, and it was easier to find what we wanted when we wanted, no matter how tired we were, and nothing was missed because we had a ready reckoner reminder implanted into the system design in case we missed something.

In short, we inadvertently stumbled across the following logic process with significant Lean implications.

LOGIC PROCESS

What you have
Plus
What you do
Equals
What you get.

This means that every step is designed to intimately and easily lead to the correct outcome.

And since one of our early mantras was

'Futility is process dismissive of outcome',

we figured we had a pretty powerful strategy developing.

Interestingly enough, all of what we have just related is really quite wordy.

So we simplified even the words we used. It came down to this:

In order to develop an intelligent process

you need NEXT STEP THINKING
underpinned by the engineering of:
SYSTEMS UNC0MPL3XITY.

Now, I know you're going to laugh at my use of silly words but let me tell you this:

When I explain all this in simple language to the next nurse I meet, they will understand exactly what I mean.

And they will be able to enact my two simple ideas:

Systems Unc0mpl3xity;
and
Next Step Thinking.

But they won't for the life of them remember anything I say about Lean Methodologies or Six Sigma.

Because no matter how simply I put it, it will all sound too complex.

And they'll already be thinking, after the first three words I say, about all the things they have to do in the next hour that will get in the way of their desperate need for caffeine.

However, they will be able to fully describe our ridiculously worded concept to any colleague they speak to in that rare moment of tranquillity we call a coffee break:

Systems Unc0mpl3xity
and
Next Step Thinking
equals
Smarter, Better, Safer.

Lastly, Dr Peter Pronovost at Johns Hopkins has made his fortune and fame on the back of a simple checklist which is useful for making sure central line insertions happen as they are supposed to happen with all the safety systems in check.

Being nurses, John and I won't be making our fortunes on anything. However, we believe we have created something equally significant and complementary to Peter Pronovost's checklist.

I call it, 'The blind side of the checklist'.

It's like the wine list that should go with every good meal.

The blind side of the checklist is this:

Everything which has a specific purpose is set out for that purpose in a way that makes it impossible to have too much or too little. Just enough to get the job done in the balance of probabilities, and set out in the order they will be used.

Nothing hidden, nothing extra.

Just the stuff you need, at hand, well displayed and ready to go.

Not because we want to be nice to our fellow nurses, but because since our managers, our patients and their lawyers are going to insist on us using an algorithm and checklist, *we* are going to insist that we are *not* going to be interrupted from successful task completion by succumbing to a chaotic failure of simple human factors and ergonomics.

I used to make a point of taking my students to the Cardiac Arrest Trolley.

We would look at the design of the trolley and discuss the Code Blue algorithm.

Then we would try to find the things we needed in order to execute that algorithm.

In particular, things got very messy when we got to the Adrenaline.

There was a drawer full of ampoules.

Our pharmacy refused to stock pre-filled syringes because they were too expensive and went out of date too quickly.

The clutter made it difficult for the students to find the one drug they truly needed, and when they did manage to find it, they still had to track down the syringes, the drawing up needle and the saline.

So we had an algorithm designed to improve the flow and effectiveness of treatment in a cardiac arrest, and a trolley designed to be as confusing as possible.

Not very smart, and not very reassuring for a junior nurse who, at any time, might be thrust into the middle of exactly such a situation *and* expected to perform to a high standard.

When the student found the adrenaline, I would say:

'Now, forget all the other drugs. They are just there to distract you away from the one thing you truly want.'

Then I would instruct them to crack the adrenaline, draw it up, and label it.

'There! Well done! In an arrest, that is exactly what you have to do.

'Even before it is asked for, draw it up and label it and sit it on a clean tray.

'When the dose is delivered, draw up another one because the chances are they are going to need it, and when they ask for it, they are going to want it. *Stat!*

'Sit the used adrenaline syringe in a dirty tray, so that at the end, when it comes to summing up, you know exactly how much was given.'

The practice demystified the action and removed, in part, the terror.

Together we created muscle memory by enacting each step with the exact presentation of the exact equipment in real time.

Improving functionality means students don't feel lost and useless. They also learn that getting 'the shakes' is a perfectly normal human response to high pressure situations, but eventually they will learn to control them.

Worried about the cost? Man! It's an investment in the future, an educational expense.

A small step on the journey towards stress inoculation.

A barrier to unnecessary deaths.

And future lawsuits.

Take it out of my pay.

DEVELOPING NEW PATHWAYS

Learning to create culture change is the same as the process of learning new skills to the point of mastery and stress inoculation.

It is about creating the internal and external environment which allows neural pathways to be generated and which will embed the new skill into muscle memory.

People learn with all kinds of brains.

We each have our own dyspraxia when it comes to fear in learning, which is why creating an environment of support and trust is so important.

Thus we have taken an age old construct and tweaked it with our own shared and accumulated wisdom.

It is basically a stress inoculation sandwich where the filling is simply the character strengths of passion, patience, practice and perseverance.

In healthcare, we all have the motivation and the aptitude to happily apply these.

We also understand that these four pillars of strength are underpinned by an appreciation of the finer details of the specific techniques of the task we are setting about learning.

We also understand that mastery of the correct technique goes through several different phases:

1. First we have the passion to observe.
2. Then we have the patience to develop a sound cognitive map.
3. Then we apply that learning in safe, optimal conditions.
4. After that we commence our journey of persistence, improving our ergonomic flow and committing our new skill to daily practice.
5. Lastly, we test our ability under high pressure conditions until we have faith that we can stringently focus and attain the desired result in the emergency setting.
6. Finally, we have the passion, again, to finely tune our learning until we have mastery of the new skill, and we become a mentor to others.

Dr Tim Leeuwenberg says:

'Take a deep breath to steady your hand.'

And this is great advice.

But what you are really doing is pausing a moment to trust.

Trust in yourself, and trust in those around you,
trust that what you observe,
what you want to happen,
the supportive environment,
and the process of unfolding the event according to the script,
are all and the one thing.

It is not enough to know what to do.

It is not enough to magically think that everyone can mindread and instinctively knows how to act.

The trust comes from the ability to communicate with and work as a team to get that knowledge happening on the ground.

It requires team training. It doesn't happen by chance.

Thus the bread in our sandwich is Trust and Technique, and what makes it tasty is the filling of passion, patience, practice and perseverance.

The magic of the operating theatre doesn't happen on its own.

It takes a diverse, multidisciplinary team.

And it takes time and effort to attain and maintain peak performance.

Use the sandwich, and whatever you have for lunch will taste superb!

HUMAN FACTORS

Do you have any LEGO®?

It might seem like a strange question, but bear with me.

This book *is* about applying creative thinking to clinical problem solving. I can still hear my colleagues saying ...

'Oh dear. What's Pete up to *now*?'

Fear not. As crazy as you think it may be in the beginning, all I'm doing is applying game thinking to entrenched problems. And believe it or not the results have impressive ramifications for those brave enough to embrace their inner child.

An emergency crashes through the door.

You have five minutes' notice.

How we do what we do determines how we handle what we do.

- Task sequencing?
- Fluxing leadership?
- Divisions of labour?
- Communication pathways?
- Programmed refreshment?

The best way to tackle such an occurrence is by thinking about it beforehand.

How do we currently respond?

How could we *better* respond?

Could we improve our current game plan so that a rapid response becomes normalised, practiced, reproducible and dependable?

Could we do more with less, and at the same time expose the people engaged in doing the 'more' to less stress and less emotional turmoil?

In short, can we reduce the vicarious trauma and increase our operational antifragility simply by gaming the problem?

I'll bet all the LEGO I own on the fact that you can.

Let's explore.

First, don't blame me. Blame Pat Croskerry – he started it.

I read a paper of his in an anaesthetic journal many years ago, and what he said was fascinating. In the article, he explored the effect of human factors in the Emergency Department, and it opened my eyes to the possibilities of human factors within our own anaesthetics specialty.

The possibility was further reinforced during a recent simulation session when it again became apparent that it is not only what we know and what we do, but how we do it, that is important.

Whilst I can't reveal any details about the sim because sims are confidential, what I can do is reflect on the human factors of a probable event at any given time: the sudden arrival of a full-blown high level emergency case.

Go!

So let's imagine that it is 11 am on Christmas Day.

The team has successfully worked on a few small cases, and maybe a fractured hip or two, but then things seem to have quietened down.

They get out the Christmas cake, the chips and dips, the Christmas crackers, the pretzels and the lollies, and just as they are starting to relax, the phone rings.

The patient is on their way up from emergency.

Now!

On the anaesthetic nursing team, each declares what they are going to do and does it:

- One sets up the Level 1 Blood Warmer.
- A second sets up the transducers.
- A third sets up the intubation equipment and the anaesthetic machine.

Then they attend to tasks as they arise.

The anaesthetist *tries* to communicate to everyone, and *tries* to ensure that everything has been done.

It is a long, complex operation, but finally it's complete.

The patient goes to ICU.

The team cleans up and retires, exhausted, to cold Christmas turkey and warm cranberry sauce.

PLAN

The *Human Factors Trauma Plan* is designed to optimise Human Factors during Trauma and other high intensity surgical (often emergency) cases by fine-tuning communication pathways, role segregation and task sequentialling.

The plan also includes leadership structures and team restoration, optimising under-utilised opportunities to re-energise the team over the evolution of the operation.

Of course, this game plan is constructed for a specific, foreseeable and often-repeated event.

However, you can develop a coordinated response plan for any such crisis in your own clinical setting.

ASSEMBLING THE CORE EMERGENCY TEAM

Airway team

In the beginning there was ... the operating room, the operating table, the anaesthetic machine and the anaesthetic trolley.

Then came the anaesthetist and the anaesthetic nurse, who are in the room by allocation. If you are lucky, there may be a registrar, which is really, really cool.

The anaesthetic nurse and the anaesthetist checked the equipment at the start of the day and have established a working rapport, so they become the centre-point of the expanding team.

The anaesthetist, or the registrar (by agreement), becomes the airway specialist, and the anaesthetic nurse joins that designate and together they become the airway management team.

Here's what they work together and accomplish:

- Induction
- Intubation
- Securing the tube
- Taping the eyes
- Inserting the temperature probe
- Placing the BIS monitor
- Putting on the warming blanket
- Positioning the urinary catheter bag for easy measurement access.

Having a specific core induction and airway management team means a one-link single-line chain of communication.

Therefore there is closed loop communication with regards to needs, expectations and shared-goal strategies.

Better, there is a single focus and therefore no distraction from the task at hand.

Line Insertion Team

The second anaesthetist becomes the line insertion specialist, and the second anaesthetic nurse joins that person to create a team.

Their job, prior to and/or after induction, is to establish monitoring, then put in the drip, the arterial line and the central line if required, and also to set up the inotropic infusions:

- IV
- Arterial line
- Central line
- Syringe drivers
- Inotropic infusions

The nurse who is allocated the task of facilitating line insertion assembles and checks all equipment required for that task sequence.

Flow and focus help this process.

There is a sensitive dependence on starting conditions, and the initial conditions are helped when, amid the swirl of activity, the line insertion team can claim their real estate and work through their time-critical goals with optimised proficiency.

Once again there is a one-link single-line chain of communication.

And closed loop communication with regards to needs, expectations and shared-goal strategies.

And again, that single focus meaning no distraction from the task at hand.

Everything about the resuscitation depends on having adequate, reliable, intravenous access and arterial monitoring.

Go! Go! Go!

Critical Bleeding Team

The first nurse who is allocated this role prepares the rapid blood transfuser and assembles and checks all equipment required for the task sequence required to give copious quantities of blood.

A second nurse prepares to check the blood products as they arrive, gets them in order so that they can easily be checked off the crossmatch form, and collates the fluid balance chart.

Once again there is a one-link single-line chain of communication.

And closed loop communication with regards to needs, expectations and shared-goal strategies.

And again, that single focus meaning no distraction from the task at hand.

Giving blood, especially through a rapid infuser, is dangerous business. An incorrectly identified unit of blood or an air bolus will kill.

Timely delivery of blood products according to the critical bleeding protocol can save the day.

Blood is life, and a good blood delivery workstation makes life safer and easier for everybody.

The Runner

The runner is a go-to person. This person assists members of the core teams as required, and otherwise awaits task allocation.

Taking Charge

In amidst the chaos, a senior anaesthetist or critical care specialist walks into the room and takes in the situation then takes charge.

'Airway team:

'Are you ok?

'Do you have everything you need to execute your plan?

'Where are you up to in your plan?

'Do you need anything?

'Person X, get them what they need.'

Then:

'Line Insertion team:

'Are you ok?

'Do you have everything you need to execute your plan?

'Where are you up to in your plan?

'Do you need anything?

'Person Y, get them what they need.'

Then:

'Critical Bleeding Protocol team:

'Are you ok?

'Do you have everything you need to execute your plan?

'Where are you up to in your plan?

'Do you need anything?

'Person Z, get them what they need.'

Finally:

'Surgical team:

'Are you ok?

'Do you have everything you need to execute your plan?

'Where are you up to in you plan?

'Do you need anything?

'Scouts, get them what they need.

'Everyone not allocated a task, please step out of the room.'

In five snapshot conversations, order is established and everyone knows exactly what is going on and where they are in the plan.

It might seem strange, the idea of removing all extra people from the room, but in general, too many extra people in the room creates confusion.

- They interrupt the communication pathways.
- They cause distraction.
- They can muddy already congested access, egress and the flow of tasks.

The new strategic response, however, delivers focused accountability and task segregation.

It is easier to respond completely and comprehensively, and easier to de-escalate as task sequences become complete.

Once induction of anaesthesia is complete and the airway is secure, that team transitions into the maintenance of anaesthesia role, as they normally would.

Once the intravenous lines, the arterial line and the central venous lines are in and secured and the first blood gas is done, that team becomes redundant. Their designated job is complete.

But their next most important role is about to commence.

The blood team is in full flight; the anaesthetic team are regrouping.

An hour of frantic activity has passed.

The senior anaesthetist understands the opportunity that arises and instructs the former line insertion team to go for a break, refresh, and then come back to start giving refreshment breaks to all the other members of the team.

It is an important regrouping strategy.

Rest combats fatigue.

After four or five hours of intense concentration without rest, individual effectiveness becomes compromised.

Sadly this occurs at exactly the time everyone will be stepping up a notch in order to safely deliver the patient to ICU.

Fatigue causes errors and errors kill.

Not much use winning the battle only to lose the war.

TEAM FLUXING

Changing circumstances demand a flexible approach to any situation on the basis that changing clinical needs and changing resource availability dictate team numbers and composition.

With this in mind, the availability of optimal numbers of personnel to navigate a situation will, on occasion, occur. However, due to the nature of emergency medicine, it may well be that only one or two nurses may be available to pursue all task sets and sequences to the best of their ability.

Still, your game plan has to acknowledge and deal with those probabilities, and recognition of such potentialities aids organisational strategic decision making, like how many people to have on night duty.

Further, junior nurses have an important opportunity as the chance to be a part of such an effort is a junction on the pathway from novice to expert.

The ideal role for the learner is being the second nurse in the critical bleeding protocol team. They get to watch the swirl of seeming chaos and learn the underlying patterns within.

As they develop competencies, they can then be escalated into other roles, and because the roles are skill based and delineated, they can function well, function safely and gain intrinsic reward and work satisfaction.

In other words, they are coached to success, and gain in terms of stress inoculation. They grow, feel a part of an important team and start to glow.

In terms of recruitment, retention and resilience, it is Win! Win! Win!

Irrespective of the situation you find yourself in, we hope that this 'game plan' may assist with your thinking.

Such a plan can be applied to myriad clinical situations, not just within the operating theatre.

Play with the idea and see what you come up with.

We know you want to!

The future of systems modelling lies dead ahead.

WORK INTENSIFICATION

We've all seen the nursing memes:

'What did you do on your days off?'
'I slept.'
'For two days?'
'Yup.'

Work: Brutal. Intense. Exhausting to the guttural level.

How did it get that way?

Why does it stay that way?

Why do we accept it as the way things have to be?

What can mere clinicians do about it?

So many questions, so few answers.

The first step is to open peoples' eyes.

And if playing Tetris in the rarefied atmosphere of Mount Everest helps, then so be it.

TECTONIC PLATE TETRIS THEORY OF WORKLOAD

The original tectonic theory of workload was deduced to better quantify actual time and effort demands in the complex work environment of the operating theatre.

It was deduced, obviously, by me, because no one else is crazy enough to come up with such an idea.

John would like to call it the Tetris Theory of Workload, and I agree that there are some particularly appealing complementary metaphors going on there.

However, having walked in the Himalayas, I have seen first hand what pressure can do, and so I concede to call it the 'Tectonic Plate Tetris Theory of Workload'.

The Theory

Workload in anaesthetic nursing occurs in chunks.

These chunks are actually blocks of work associated with particular task events. They have a finite sequence of steps which, assembled in chronological order, describe the performance of an anaesthetic and, collectively, an operating list from a nurse's perspective.

Each block is unique, finite and concrete in terms of effort and time required to safely complete it.

These blocks continue to build over the course of the day, and as work intensifies beyond a certain threshold, corroding stamina and escalating workload pressures play a part in deciding the ensuing quality and safety of the performance environment.

Repeated day after day, this default work expectation becomes the inherent safety culture.

So: what does all this mean?

The first ever mud map of our theory was a mental picture of a series of stratified layers, with each layer a block compressing the one below.

Each block represents an operating theatre case with its related task- and contingency-related activities.

As the workload compounds, the ability of the clinician to deal with it becomes compromised, and so the workload then impinges on the only flexible time allocation available – that of breaks.

So workload first compresses rest periods, reducing the clinician's ability to maintain their stamina.

The next most compressible time involves low hierarchy micro and macro tasks including, for example, lower order paperwork, presence at Time-Out, hand washing, sterility and even restocking. Thus errors of omission start to occur because constraints on time do not permit full compliance with systems processes and procedural policies.

Finally, physical and cognitive function begin to erode as psychomotor exhaustion sets in.

Intensifiers:

Some factors have a multiplier effect on the size of the tectonic work plate.

For example:

- number of operations on a list
- uncontrolled variances e.g. emergency lists, with combined adult and paediatric cases
- degree of complexity
- distance from storerooms
- distance from patient pickup points
- distance from specialised equipment repositories
- accessibility to facilities and adequacy of facilities
- being on an early shift following a late shift
- fatigue-related psychomotor inefficiencies
- stock levels
- equipment
- maintenance level of equipment
- inefficient systems of work
- complexity of paperwork and data collection.

Other multipliers exist which I have failed to mention, but the above are enough to highlight that myriad intensifiers contribute to workload and thus to the magnitude of the tectonic plates which comprise each workload block.

How This Affects the Clinician

It leaves nurses feeling unable to complete all the tasks to the highest level of their competency.

Nurses begin to take short cuts to fit the work required into the time available.

Nurses begin to become critical of other nurses' abilities and indeed their 'professionalism' because the trolley or cupboards are not fully restocked.

Nurses are led away from bedside care to complete these 'non clinical duties' in order to avoid peer criticism.

Rather than saying that we are indeed unable to perform all the tasks, rather than saying to our manager that 'What you ask of us isn't sustainable, professional and repeatable in a meaningful and predictable way', we all just go about our work bitching and cussing about how we have been burdened with forever increasing levels of non-clinical work.

All to the detriment of safe clinical patient care.

The Answer

The answer to the problem is not just to consider time and motion.

It is more complex than that.

It is linked to our Diagram of Human Performance described in the next chapter, 'The Edge of Coping', where time has incorporated workload distribution and workload intensity, and motion has been replaced by human factors, ergonomics and systems processes.

The next and most important part of the diagram is psychomotor performance (comprising both cognitive science and endurance physiology).

It explores the territory of optimal human performance and, equally importantly, the endpoint of human effectiveness in relation to safely undertaking the task at hand.

Summation

The Tectonic Plate Tetris Theory of Workload proposed by Smith and Gibbs (2014) fills a void in current nursing knowledge and practice.

This void is apparent across the entire nursing profession and the healthcare industry.

It is conspicuous by its absence in consideration in any industrial agreement.

It is conspicuous by its absence in any system of work construct.

It is conspicuous by its absence in the execution of managerial knowledge.

And it is conspicuous by its absence in the performance of clinical healthcare duties.

Consideration of The Tectonic Plate Tetris Theory of Workload will aid in the delivery of high quality and safe healthcare for both the patient and the caregiver.

It will result in fewer errors, fewer near misses, lower complication rates, reduced sick leave and less conflict at work.

It will result in decreased healthcare expenditure on all of the above related indices, not just to the tune of dollars, but to the tune of hundreds of millions of dollars worldwide.

Most of the science is already there.

The quantum gap is in the recognition and application of this knowledge to healthcare.

It is said that 'To err is human'.

I would counter that with: 'To enforce conditions that ensure humans err is inhumane.'

FATIGUE

FATIGUE

Look at a nurse and describe what you see.

I see tired people who go beyond the call of duty to care for everyone but themselves.

When caring for others,
don't leave yourself behind.

This quote is from Jennifer Reidy, Compassion Fatigue, Ireland.

Great advice, Jen.

THE EDGE OF COPING

The heart is a hollow muscular organ.

It contracts and relaxes in a rhythmic, strategic fashion to pump blood around the body.

It works through a system of nerves and muscle fibres and valves and inflow and outflow tracts, all of which work together to deliver a unique, effective and efficient workload which has the capacity both to increase and decrease depending on the demands required of it, the metrics of which get relayed to it by a series of predominantly negative feedback loops.

As the heart is put under workload stress, two things become apparent.

First, it becomes increasingly important to ensure that the heart muscle has sufficient oxygenation and blood flow of its own to ensure its safe hyper-dynamic functioning.

Second, the heart's muscular wall stretches to accommodate the newly increased requirements.

Starling's Law describes the performance of the heart in relation to this increased capacitance.

As the heart wall is stretched, there comes a point beyond which the heart muscle loses its ability to pump effectively, and cardiac output starts to fall.

The heart is beyond its ability to cope with the workload demanded of it, and it starts to fail.

The range of possible solutions to this problem covers:

1. Do nothing.
2. On recognising a struggling heart, give medications which make the heart beat harder and faster.
3. Take measures to protect the heart and offload the pressures imposed on it, making the heart beat better and with less effort whilst at the same time undertaking measures to correct the underlying problem.

Doing nothing is an ostrich.

Beating it with medication is flogging a dead horse, and could easily be reframed as 'Stalin's Law'.

The third is 'Starling's Law', accepting the limits of systems sustainability, and respecting the confines of those limits.

In 2013, I was involved in creating, for the Australian College of Operating Room Nurses, a guideline for the management of fatigue.

It was a landmark step for the College, because for the first time, they recognised the negative consequences of fatigue on clinicians and on patient outcomes, and were prepared to take steps to address the problem.

Whilst participating in this process, it became obvious to me that the biggest obstacle to implementing fatigue mitigation processes was not one of evidence, because the evidence has been around for more than twenty years.

Long enough to see wide-sweeping changes in a number of other major industries.

The biggest obstacle, I saw, was a problem of mindset.

CASE STUDY #9:
COME-BY-CHANCE

Sarah, an anaesthetist, was second-on-call one weekend. She happened to wander in to see how things were going.

It had been a busy weekend and yet another operation was just commencing.

The operating theatre team looked a bit work weary and amid the fatigue there were multiple conversations going on. Her first impression was how loud the room was.

Sarah could see the anaesthetic registrar, Bianca, was having trouble inserting an arterial line whilst struggling to also keep an eye on the anaesthetic monitor. Arterial lines can be tricky at the best of times, the least part being trying to thread the 20G catheter over the tiny wire whilst maintaining a sterile field.

Sarah called, 'Below Ten Thousand'.

Quiet descended on the room allowing Bianca to better concentrate.

She suddenly got good arterial blood flow, advanced the wire, then the cannula, and with relief attached the tubing and secured the line.

'Thank you, everybody. You can stand down now,' she sighed with relief.

'Well done,' Sarah told Bianca. 'Now go for a cuppa whilst I look after things here. You've certainly earned a break!'

Mindset problems are difficult to see from within until they are pointed out to us.

The first mindset problem is that our social contract is stacked against us:

We adhere to the concept that that, as clinical nurses, we will do anything asked of us in the interests of meeting others' needs.

Don't blame yourself for that skewed perspective. Game Theory Mathematics and the 'Mathematics of Burnout' explain that people who are meaningfully invested in their work are statistically unlikely to say no to any request asked of them, if the answer of 'no' means that a third, often unknown, party is likely to suffer.

It's part of the utility payoff equation.

Secondly, we have to realise that, as a cohort, we really don't get time to 'think'.

To be fair, not even non-frantic people take the time, and effort, to think,

To quote a Greek philosopher, Diogenes:

People give money to beggars who are lame and blind,
because they can always imagine a time
when they themselves
may lose an eye or a leg.
But they never give money to a philosopher,
because they can never imagine a time
when they may be required to think.

For one hundred years we have laboured under the workplace performance mantra of time and motion.

For nurses it means:

- If there's still time, for God's sake, do something!
- It is a workplace methodology which feels right.
- It gets things done with a minimum of cognitive input and a maximum of delegation.

No one stops to wonder if the person being delegated to is busy.

It is assumed by proxy that they still have room in their diary to do 'more' than the 'more' that the delegator doesn't have time to do and so delegates.

So time and motion as a methodology feels good, is simple, reassuring, authoritative ... and wrong.

It is wrong not because it is wholly wrong, but because, as proof of the dual processing theory of the mind, we stopped thinking too soon.

It leaves out the most essential component of human performance:

Humanity.

Or, to be more specific, psychomotor performance.

Time

Just like so much else, time is a resource.

There is only so much of it.

Time for us is a factor in considering the usage limits of:

- infrastructure
- equipment
- and human capital.

There is only so much of everything to go around, and

only so much time to use each in, each of which takes ... time.

Therefore, the summative time, whether you use these things in series or in parallel, has an upper, concrete, mathematical limit.

We are used to seeing time as flexible, and we make it appear flexible by compressing it and creating a so-called time pressure.

Though we know that pressure, real and perceived, past a certain point, degrades performance and decision making.

In terms of human capital, time seems compressible because you can make people work harder and faster.

You can add in layers of extra tasks, otherwise known as work intensification, and you can impinge on non-productive time, AKA tea breaks, lunch breaks and finishing times ... and it always seems to fit.

For each little bit you add in, you can always use the same rationalisation:

'But it only takes a second!'

Pete's Rule of Workload:

The simplest way to determine if Work exceeds the current capacity of the resource to deal with it is if you got your breaks, and if you got home on time.

So in terms of human capital, time is, in fact, concrete.

We just make it 'seem' elastic by disrespecting the boundaries of our most valuable resources, our infrastructure, our equipment ... and most of all, our people.

Time factors of workload can further be divided into workload distribution and work intensity.

Workload distribution is the distribution of work over the course of your shift.

Work intensity occurs when workload distribution is skewed in time.

So you get busier and busier as your day progresses and your task load piles up.

The problem is that we as nurses haven't had a way to visualise this problem.

Until now.

The Tectonic Plate Tetris Theory of Workload came about on a day just like many other days.

We were being smashed with monotonous regularity and some quite nasty conflict was resulting because of it.

So I took it upon myself to try to work out why.

I mean, I know it's not hard to figure out why, but what I wanted to know was: *why* why?

What lessons were we repeatedly ignoring to perpetuate an unsafe work environment?

I used a journey mapping app to record each task sequence I performed over the course of the day.

What I found astonished even me:

- Eighty-six task sequences, some simple, many complex, amid the unstructured, confused and convoluted evolution of a standard run of the mill weekend emergency and semi-urgent operating list day.
- Six and a half minutes per task sequence.

Crazy!

- Late lunch and only time for a wee break and a glass of water in the afternoon.

Stupid.

- Fourteen errors of omission in care.

Frightening.

Fortunately, none were potentially fatal. And, to be kind, it was an early shift after a late shift, so I had worked at a frantic pace for 19 hours in 28, all on five hours' sleep.

What I realised in recording my day was that I could render my task sequences into discrete blocks of activity.

Each took a fairly predictable amount of time, and each was sequenced one after another.

And I realised that as the day progressed, all the blocks started smashing together.

Like tectonic plates.

In amongst my observations was the revelation that, being discrete blocks, I could see where the leverage points existed to offset the cascade by using more effective resourcing and decision making algorithms, and also where it was possible to provide a safety net of rest and restoration, should appropriate systems allow, enabling me to refresh and recharge my energy levels before the inevitable fatigue led irrevocably to the inevitability of errors.

I ran this past my friend and colleague, John Gibbs, and he thought it looked like Tetris.

But I've walked the Himalayas, and I've seen what pressure can do, so we agreed to call it the Tectonic Plate Tetris Theory of Workload.

You can see what I mean.

First go the micro-tasks.

Then go your rest breaks.

Then goes safety as formalised policies and procedures are made inactionable, become eroded and succumb to production pressure.

Time is fixed.

It is not elastic, even if we make it seem so.

Motion

Motion is how we do what we do.

If you want a definition of a 'rut', it is this:

> *Always doing what we do*
> *because that's the way we've always done it*
> *with the expectation of a different outcome.*

It's not that the work isn't doable.

It's that it is not doable from within our current systems of work.

As work exceeds the availability of time to do it, the system descends into unsustainability and chaos.

And in the presence of chaos, it takes so much more energy to focus on your own little part in the whole cyclone.

As workload descends into chaos, the Cynefin framework offers some useful observations:

- When things are simple, you engage, step by step.
- When things get complicated, you probe, developing a hierarchy of prioritised actions, and you set about achieving your goals.

- When things become complex, you strategise by contingency. Your Plan B becomes your Plan A, and you develop a new Plan B.
- You prioritise the things you must do, and let go of the things that would simply be 'good to do'.
- When things descend into chaos, you do 'anything'.

And believe me. You will.

Cynefin is not a strategy.

It is a workload-specific cautionary tale.

If you want to look at motion as an entity, here are some components:

There's human factors and ergonomics:

- the positioning of everything, and the twists and turns and strains and traffic movements and load distributions you have to go through to accomplish your tasks.
- Ease is good.

Then there's systems processes, both real and imagined:

- 'Real' is how you perform the systems.
- 'Imagined' is how they are written in the procedure manual.

Built into this is complexity:

- Policies upon policies and tasks upon tasks which, when put together, overload you beyond your ability to comply effectively with them, given the time you have to do them in.

Maybe it is now time to incorporate into nurse/patient ratios the concept of work/futility ratios!

How much of your day is spent clearing obstacles from your care plan, like getting orders written, chasing results and waiting for someone else to do something so that you can do your thing?

The current nurse work/futility ratio is somewhere between 30% and 50%.

So instead of platitudes that fly in the face of human nature and become your new prison because they are repeated and reinforced and grow to form beliefs, how about we accept the reality of our limitations, and expect ourselves to be no more than human?

Motion is all about flow.

It is about sequencing work.

And developing systems which aid flow, implementing pre-formed layers of contingencies which, when enacted, resource or constrain the chaos.

Integrating time and motion means that you can only do so much, and expect to do it well and sustainably.

We can do more, but the risk is enormous and the possible consequences unconscionable.

So if you want a system to work hard, and it seems we can't help ourselves but demand it of healthcare, optimising the way we think about and construct process becomes critical.

High performance team methodologies set about optimising the system.

We consider motion to be fixed, immutable.

But it is the one thing in this whole equation that is flexible.

It is the one thing that can change to bring the fatigue

picture back into high performance, high reliability safety and quality alignment.

Performance

Humans do nursing. That is why we look at human performance.

If we were robots, we would be looking at mechanical stress points.

Psychomotor performance is comprised of cognitive and endurance performance.

Cognitive Performance

- Rest
- Nutrition and fluid maintenance
- Well constructed planning and contingency management
- Alertness
- Cognitive load
- Distraction
- Checklists and memory aids
- Building strong neural pathways
- Unburdening

Endurance Performance

- Rest
- Nutrition and fluid maintenance
- Well constructed workflows
- Alertness
- Muscle load
- Proprioception
- Mechanical aids

- Building muscle memory
- Unburdening

We know a lot about these.

We know when and how the brain functions best (when it is rested and fed and not overloaded).

We know when and how the body functions best (when it is rested and fed and not overloaded).

Then add to this emotion:

We know when and how emotions function best (when we have time for defusing, processing and disentangling).

We just refuse to apply that knowledge to ourselves.

And we consider psychomotor performance parameters to be flexible whereas, in order to be high performance, boundaries appear which are concrete and definitive.

Beyond these limits, performance is degraded.

Therefore, the only thing that is flexible in performance is the level of performance you can deliver given the constraints you suffer in real time.

High performance or low performance.

It is systems-imposed, and the result is out of your hands.

Why should we worry about this?

In 1992, preventable deaths from medical errors, in Australia alone, were calculated at 14,000. That is the equivalent of 26 of the world's largest planes (built in three-class configuration) being flown into the ground.

In a single, smallish country.

In one year.

If you believe the Institute of Medicine's 'To Err is Human' report, 50% of these deaths could be said to be directly attributable to fatigue.

This is the biggest untreated epidemic in healthcare today.

To put it on a scale:

- The number of people diagnosed with bowel cancer in Australia is 14,000 per year.
- The cost of treating bowel cancer in 2011 was $1 billion dollars.
- The happy result of treating bowel cancer in 2011 was a five year survival rate of 66%.

The five-year survival rate for death through preventable medical error?

Zero.

So, putting it all together around Starling's Law, this is what we get.

The more you push a system beyond the point of sustainability, the more likely it is to fall over.

The heart is subject to not only time and motion factors, but performance pressures as well.

And most critical to sustained performance is coronary artery blood flow, or how the heart nourishes and restores itself.

If it is true for the heart, then it is true for yourself as well, as a dynamic person within a dynamic system within a dynamic organisation.

The system should be robust enough to allow you to drop an average person into it and have them perform well.

Currently, we stick imperfect people in an imperfect system. And expect them to be perfect.

If we link the three elements together, we get the edges of workload performance, outside which systems failure occurs.

- If we link time and motion, we get the Edge of Sustainability.
- If we link motion and performance, we get the Edge of Doability.
- If we link performance and time, we get the Edge of Coping.

Outside these we get fatigue, musculoskeletal injury and stress.

Inside, we get

- optimised safety
- optimised outcome and
- optimised engagement.

So if this is you …

If this is the dot point singularity of you existing with this workload construct, this pyramid of human work performance, what are your rights, your responsibilities and your duties of care?

Your rights

Workplace Health and Safety Legislation gives you the right to a safe workplace in terms of both physical and psychological health.

Your Responsibilities

Refer specifically to your professional registration.

Practising in ways which comply with Accreditation Standards, wherein is included the Governance of Safety.

Layered over this is the patient's right to receive safe care.

Then there are your duties of care:

- to yourself
- to your family
- to your patients
- to your fellow staff members.

Now I wonder ...

What is your agreed social contract? And who agreed to what? Did your employer representatives, and let's be clear – an employer representative is a person (e.g. Squizzy Square) with authority and presumably accountability, and you have power against a person, as opposed to an employer (e.g. Oblong Hospital), which is an abstract entity, against which you have no power –

Did your employer representatives, upon you signing your employment contract, in the back of their minds, think:

'This person agrees to work beyond the edge of sustainability, beyond the edge of doability, and beyond the edge of coping?'

And did you, upon signing your employment contract, in the back of your mind, think:

'I agree to work at the level of optimised sustainability, optimised outcomes, and optimised engagement ... because that is where I *really* would like to be?'

Did you, in other words, agree, or not agree, to work ad infinitum within a *sick system* of *work*, where it can be the toss of a coin between being a competent survivor, a demoralised burn-out victim, or, over time, possibly both, all because a passive person, rather than advocating on your behalf, somewhere, somehow, offloads an unsustainable workload onto you and offloads the blame onto an abstract entity?

Of course, sometimes you will be asked to dig *very* deep into your reserves in order to get the job done.

But that should be the exception, not the rule.

And the risk-benefit ratio with respect to the outcome should be worth it.

Legendary actions should remain legendary because of their uncommonality.

How we think about fatigue

How we think about fatigue can be demonstrated using the dual processing theory of the brain.

Let me show you.

I'm in Lorne for the day with the family, and because we like beach cricket, I go to buy a beach cricket ball because, silly me, I only remembered the bat.

I go into the shop, and there it is, a bat and ball set ... for $1:10.

I say to the shopkeeper, 'I really only want the ball.'

He says, 'Well, I suppose I could, sell you the ball, but together, the bat and ball cost $1.10. If I sell them separately, the bat costs a dollar more than the ball.'

So how much is the ball?

You see, that is the way we think about fatigue.

Our brains trick us into deciding on one easy answer,

and that answer, although it is often wrong, is very hard to get out of our heads.

Our brains say, 'I survived. I coped. Just. I don't have the energy to worry about it now. So I'll worry about it *next* time.'

But when it comes to next time, our brains say the same thing.

Five cents.

So how can we change that?

We need to give you a new frame of reference.

How many of you know how to make a fly?

I once bought a textbook on how a fly is made. It went into a lot of detail, mostly on genetics and technique.

How many of you know how to *kill* a fly?

The instruction manual on how to kill a fly is a mere three sentences long.

Your Policy and Procedures Manual is a manual on how to create fatigue. It is supremely detailed and complex. Encyclopaedic, in fact.

The ACORN Position Statement is four pages long. It contains the instructions needed to kill fatigue.

You don't have to know everything about everything to solve the problem.

You only have to know what *you* can do for *yourself.*

Start in ever-increasing concentric circles centred ... about ... yourself. Know your own limits:

- 17 hours of wakefulness equates to a performance equivalent of a blood alcohol reading of 0.05

- 12.5 hours of work increases the rate of error by 200–300%
- Know the IM SAFE acronym, and know how to calculate your sleep debt.
- Use FAWPI to identify how your fatigue is affecting you, and use it to communicate that to those who can't possibly understand.

And advocate to everyone around you, family, peers, managers, what you know about the risks, personal and professional, of fatigue in nursing.

So in conclusion

Because there is not enough time, we don't give ourselves the chance to think about time or motion or human performance.

Somehow, we need a circuit breaker which allows us to disentangle, to step back, to clear the muddy pools of the mind and allow clarity to give us the embarrassingly simple answers to the problem we have overburdened ourselves with for so long.

In a humanistic profession we are only human and being human, we should construct our work to fit us and our needs, rather than contort ourselves to fit the work so often, so heavily layered upon us.

We want to obey Starling's law. Not Stalin's law.

FATIGUE
AS A WORKPLACE INJURY
(FAWPI)

We at Below Ten Thousand have invented a whole new quantum assessment paradigm for the field of fatigue research.

We call it the 'FAWPI'.

FAWPI is a virtual, virtual currency invented to subjectively quantify and qualify levels of fatigue in the individual.

It is more interesting than the Verbal Analogue Scale and more fun than the Likert scale.

Until now, nurses have had no ability to offer a qualitative or quantitative analysis to accurately describe how they are feeling when, at times of fatigue intoxication, analytical cognition is reduced.

FAWPI offers a simple descriptive application which may be analytically deconstructed once cognitive function is restored by rest.

Further, whilst 'others' may fail to appreciate expressions of fatigue due to suspended belief arising from an inability to comprehend vague perspectival narratives, application of FAWPI may offer a tool for increased mutual understanding by providing a simple, transmissible and easily articulated symbol of some speculative value.

Whilst FAWPI is not yet validated as a scientific tool nor as a virtual, virtual currency, it goes a small way to providing raw data pertaining to the level of physical and mental fatigue that is being suffered by an individual and which on further examination and analysis may yield a pathway to deeper understanding of the phenomenon that is occurring.

Industry-wide use of FAWPI may yet yield a critical mass of data which may reveal, for the first time, a stark and visual realisation of the tsunami of fatigue currently inundating clinical health professionals as they struggle to cope with overwhelming demand in the face of underwhelming clinical infrastructure, time and human resources.

To get an indication of relative value, the metaphorical exchange rate for a FAWPI is:

$$1 \; FAWPI = 1 \; AUD$$

And the 1–1000 FAWPI scale represents, in broad terms, how much you would pay to be able to reset your fatigue debt to zero right now.

If 1000 FAWPI seem like too much, then maybe it's a long time since you fell asleep waiting for the lights to change whilst driving home from work.

HOW TO USE FAWPI

Zero FAWPI
- I'm good.
- Laugh with me.

10 FAWPI
- Yeah …
- I'm ok.
- Just give me coffee.

100 FAWPI

- Tired.
- Can think but needs caution.
- I can feel my thermoregulation getting scrambled.
- Double checking of the self commences.
- Give me the rest of the day off.

300 FAWPI

- Zombie territory.
- Can hardly move.
- Can hardly think.
- Still pleasant, but ...
- Probably aching all over.
- Best just leave me alone, I think.
- In 24 hours I'll feel better.

500 FAWPI

- Zombie and mad.
- Dangerous.
- Stay away or I'll rip your head off.
- Cooling off period required!
- I could use three days' sleep!
- And *don't you dare* interrupt me!

1000 FAWPI

- Destruction of the soul.
- Dead tired.
- Asleep at the wheel, and I don't care.
- Give me a week's holiday, you bastard.
- Better still, make it a month.
- *Now!!!!!!*

Disclaimer: FAWPI is an acronym which symbolises the physical, physiological, psychological, cognitive, emotional and existential expression of fatigue in subjective increments.

FAWPI has no cash value, and is not tradable as a monetary, fiscal, economic or barter form of exchange. If you are after money, look someplace else.

IM SAFE

The biggest paradox in the provision of healthcare is fatigue.

Fatigue comes from production pressure, the need to provide care 24/7 in contravention of human circadian rhythms, and the economic desire to have the minimum number of people provide the maximum amount of care.

In 1994, Dawson and Reid published the paper 'Fatigue, alcohol and performance impairment' which found a correlation between fatigue, intoxication and performance. (see: https://www.nature.com/articles/40775).

Healthcare, however, has steadfastly refused to change, to the suffering of patients and clinicians alike.

And whilst each hospital has a drug and alcohol policy which imposes bans on staff attending work whilst intoxicated, they make attendance whilst under the influence of fatigue intoxication not only permissible but a condition of continued employment.

The easy, social and timely answer is simple:

Make the drug and alcohol policy an intoxication policy and include fatigue as a cause of intoxication.

The rationale is that drugs, alcohol *and* fatigue similarly erode performance beyond well-established thresholds.

If 17 hours of wakefulness equates to a performance equivalent of a blood alcohol reading of 0.05, then work hours should be arranged so that staff members are removed from clinical decision making and safely off the road by the time they could reasonably be presumed to have been awake for 17 hours.

The worst time to make a sound decision or judgement is at a time when your ability to make a sound decision or judgement is impaired.

Self-awareness is unreliable.

If self-assessed performance was reliable, no one would ever get caught over the limit whilst driving.

The airline industry upholds an IM SAFE acronym.

If an employee is affected by:

- **I**llness
- **M**edication
- **S**leep deprivation or stress
- **A**lcohol
- **F**atigue, or
- **E**motion

then they should excuse themselves from duty.

The implications for healthcare are huge, but the first step is to decide to act.

Once the decision to act is made, the solutions will become apparent.

All that is then required is that we must have the will and the fortitude to embrace those solutions.

SUMMATION:
THE BELOW TEN THOUSAND
WAY TO CLINICIAN-LED
CULTURE CHANGE

If you have made it this far, you are totally awesome, totally cool, and if we ever get sick, we want you as our nurse!

The upshot of this text is that a lot of people are going to hate it, because the one thing that will get in the road of nurses eating their young is nurses developing the emotional intelligence that will see them taking care of their own needs as fastidiously as they take care of their patients' needs.

Nurses have a lot to give. Our work demands we give all we can, and then some.

The expectations should be a meeting of the minds about a rational norm that prevents harm to staff and therefore prevents harm to patients.

There is no magic. There is no luck. There is only professionalism. Hopefully this text will help you help others bring more professionalism into your work life.

John and I wish you a brilliant life and an empowering career. That is our wish for all nurses, and why I wrote this book.

Take care out there!

Pete Smith

ROB'S
TOP TEN
FURTHER READING

1. A PATHWAY TO CLINICIAN-LED CULTURE CHANGE IN THE OPERATING THEATRE

Author(s): Gibbs, J.; Smith, P.

Source: Journal of Perioperative Practice; Jun 2016; vol. 26 (no. 6); p. 134-137
Publication Date: Jun 2016
Publication Type(s): Academic Journal

Abstract:

Noise in the operating theatre environment has remained a persistent and unresolved problem (Szalma & Hancock 2011). The problem currently lacks an effective solution (Schafer et al 2012). In order to partially resolve this issue, the authors created a behavioural noise reduction tool called 'Below Ten Thousand'. This study identifies a potential solution to the problem of behavioural noise in the operating theatre and indicates further research must be undertaken to identify the full scale of benefits this technique can deliver to the team environment in the operating theatre.

Database: CINAHL

2. 'BELOW TEN THOUSAND': AN EFFECTIVE BEHAVIOURAL NOISE REDUCTION STRATEGY?

Author(s): Smith, Pete; Gibbs, John

Source: ACORN: The Journal of Perioperative Nursing in Australia; Sep 2016; vol. 29 (no. 3); p. 29-32
Publication Date: Sep 2016
Publication Type(s): Academic Journal

Available at ACORN: The Journal of Perioperative Nursing in Australia from EBSCO (CINAHL Plus with Full Text)

Database: CINAHL

3. EAST LANCASHIRE HOSPITAL TRUST CREATES AN OPEN CULTURE PAVING THE WAY FOR SERVICE IMPROVEMENT 'BELOW TEN THOUSAND'

Author(s): Tomlinson, Robert

Source: Journal of Perioperative Practice; May 2018; vol. 28 (no. 5); p. 115-119

Publication Date: May 2018

Publication Type(s): Academic Journal

Abstract:

Reacting to a never event is difficult and often embarrassing for staff involved. East Lancashire Hospitals NHS Trust has demonstrated that treating staff with respect after a never event, creates an open culture that encourages problem solving and service improvement. The approach has allowed learning to be shared and paved the way for the trust to be the first in the UK to launch the patient centric behavioural noise reduction strategy 'Below ten thousand'.

Database: CINAHL

4. 14000 PREVENTABLE DEATHS IN AUSTRALIAN HOSPITALS

Source: BMJ

Publication date: June 1995:

Location: https://doi.org/10.1136/bmj.310.6993.1487

Cite this as: BMJ 1995;310:1487

An official report on Australia's hospital system shows that tens of thousands of patients die of, or become permanently disabled as a result of, preventable causes after admission. Preliminary findings of a study commissioned by the federal health department estimate that between 10000 and 14000 people died of preventable causes in both public and private hospitals in 1992. In addition, between 25000 and 30000 people experienced a preventable adverse event that led to permanent disability of some kind.

The Australian hospital care study found that preventable disabilities occurred in 1% of hospital admissions and deaths in 0.5% of admissions.

5. ADVERSE EFFECT OF NOISE IN THE OPERATING THEATRE ON SURGICAL-SITE INFECTION

Author(s): Kurmann, A; Peter, M; Tschan, F; Mühlemann, K; Candinas, D; Beldi, G

Source: The British journal of surgery; Jul 2011; vol. 98 (no. 7); p. 1021-1025

Publication Date: Jul 2011

Publication Type(s): Research Support, Non-U.S. Gov't Journal Article

PubMedID: 21618484

Available at The British Journal of Surgery from Wiley Online Library Medicine and Nursing Collection 2018 – NHS

Abstract:

BACKGROUND: The aim of this pilot study was to evaluate the noise level in an operating theatre as a possible surrogate marker for intraoperative behaviour, and to detect any correlation between sound level and subsequent surgical-site infection (SSI).

METHODS: The sound level was measured during 35 elective open abdominal procedures. The noise intensity was registered digitally in decibels (dB) every second. A standard questionnaire was used to evaluate the behaviour of the surgical team during the operation. The primary outcome parameter was the SSI rate within 30 days of surgery.

RESULTS: The overall rate of SSI was six of 35 (17 per cent). Demographic parameters and duration of operation were not significantly different between patients with, or without SSI. The median sound level (43.5 (range 26.0-60.0) versus 25.0 (25.0-60.0) dB; $P = 0.040$) and median level above baseline

(10·7 (0·6-33·3) versus 0·6 (0·5-10·8); P = 0·001) were significantly higher for patients who developed a SSI.

The sound level was at least 4 dB above the median in 22·5 per cent of the peaks in patients with SSI compared with 10·7 per cent in those without (P = 0·029). Talking about non-surgery-related topics was associated with a significantly higher sound level (P = 0·024).

CONCLUSION: Intraoperative noise volume was associated with SSI. This may be due to a lack of concentration, or a stressful environment, and may therefore represent a surrogate parameter by which to assess the behaviour of a surgical team.

Database: Medline

6. INTERRUPTIONS AND DISTRACTIONS IN THE GYNAECOLOGICAL OPERATING THEATRE: IRRITATING OR DANGEROUS?

Author(s): Yoong, Wai; Khin, Ayemon; Ramlal, Navin; Loabile, Bogadi; Forman, Stephen

Source: Ergonomics; 2015; vol. 58 (no. 8); p. 1314-1319

Publication Date: 2015

Publication Type(s): Journal Article Observational Study

PubMedID: 25672986

Abstract:

Distractions and interference can include visual (e.g. staff obscuring monitors), audio (e.g. noise, irrelevant communication) and equipment problems. Level of distraction is usually defined as I: relatively inconsequential; II: > one member of the surgical team affected; III: the entire surgical team affected.

The aim of this study was to observe the frequency and impact of distracting events and interruptions on elective gynaecology cases. Data from 35 cases were collected from 10 consecutive operating sessions. Mean number of interruptions was 26 episodes/case, while mean number of level II/III distractions was 17 episodes/case.

Ninety per cent of interruptions occur in the first 30 minutes of the procedure and 80.9% lead to level II/III distraction. Although no complications were directly attributable to the observed distractions, the mean prolongation of operating time was 18.46 minutes/case.

Understanding their effects on theatre environment enables appropriate measures to be taken so that theatre productivity and patient safety are optimised.

PRACTITIONER SUMMARY: This observational study of 35 elective cases shows a mean interruption rate of 26 episodes/case with 80.9% affecting > one member of operating team, leading to mean prolongation of 18.46 minutes/case. Theatre staff should be aware of these findings and appropriate measures taken to optimise theatre productivity and patient safety.

Database: Medline

7. VARIATIONS IN NON-TECHNICAL SKILLS IN EMERGENCY AND ELECTIVE THEATRES - A PROSPECTIVE STUDY

Author(s): O'Kelly J.; Ip B.; Paisley A.

Source: International Journal of Surgery; Nov 2015; vol. 23

Publication Date: Nov 2015

Publication Type(s): Conference Abstract

Abstract:

AIM: To assess the non-technical skills of surgeons in emergency versus elective theatre settings. To evaluate the use and compliance to the 'sterile cockpit' during critical situations. Methods: 9 emergency and 8 elective procedures were observed at a large teaching hospital. The non-technical skills of the primary operator were assessed during the pre-list brief and throughout each operation. A standardised NOTSS checklist was used to document positive and negative behaviours against four behavioural categories. Critical periods were noted, and whether the operator opened the 'sterile cockpit', recognised by theatre staff, and what the noise in the theatre during that time was. RESULTS: Positive behaviours are less prevalent in the emergency setting (Emergency 146/177 opportunities versus elective 154/165 P = 0.003), and negative behaviours are more prevalent (15/246, 0/216 P = 0.019). Communication is poorer in the emergency setting. There is no significant difference in opening of the sterile cockpit or in the background noise during critical periods between the two settings (Elective 65dB, emergency 68.3dB P = 0.1399). Conclusion: Non-technical skills are poorer in the emergency setting, particularly the theatre brief and communication. The sterile field is rarely opened formally but there is no difference in noise levels between the settings.

Database: EMBASE

8. CAN WE HEAR OURSELVES THINK? AN OBSERVATIONAL STUDY OF NOISE AND INTERRUPTIONS IN THE OPERATING THEATRE

Author(s): Clancy C.; Bukhari Y.; Joyce M.

Source: Irish Journal of Medical Science; Sep 2013; vol. 182 (no. 7)

Publication Date: Sep 2013

Publication Type(s): Conference Abstract

Available at Irish Journal of Medical Science from EBSCO (MEDLINE Complete)

Abstract:

INTRODUCTION: There are many factors which can interfere with performance during critical or complicated stages of any procedure. Surgeon related factors such as fatigue and stress combined with physical factors such as lighting and noise may affect surgical outcomes. Optimising the operating theatre environment may avoid surgical error and adverse events. The Sterile Cockpit Rule in the aviation industry forbids, by law, all non-essential activities and conversations by cabin crew and pilots during critical phases of flight as studies have shown these impair pilot performance. There is, however, a paucity of information regarding noise levels in the operating theatre. The aim of this study is to identify and quantify potential sources of distraction and noise.

METHODS: An independent observer recorded potential distractions in minor, intermediate and major surgical procedures throughout a range of specialities. The incidence of irrelevant conversation, door opening, bleepers intercom/ phone ringing and cleaning/stocking were recorded on a pre-designed pro-forma to assist homogeneity of data collection. Interruptions were recorded from skin incision to closure. All conversations related to the current surgery and teaching activities were excluded. Results: 50 operations were observed (10 laparoscopic). Length of operation ranged from 20-240 min. There was an average of 25 irrelevant conversations (3.6 per 10 min), 11 bleeps/intercom/phone (1.7 per 10 min) and door opening occurred an average of 25 times (3.5 per 10 min).

CONCLUSIONS: A significant reduction in the number of potentially distracting factors may be possible within the operating theatre which could lead to improved surgical outcomes.

Database: EMBASE

9. CRITICAL PHASE DISTRACTIONS IN ANAESTHESIA AND THE STERILE COCKPIT CONCEPT

Author(s): Broom, M A; Capek, A L; Carachi, P; Akeroyd, M A; Hilditch, G

Source: Anaesthesia; Mar 2011; vol. 66 (no. 3); p. 175-179

Publication Date: Mar 2011

Publication Type(s): Journal Article

PubMedID: 21320085

Available at Anaesthesia from Wiley Online Library
Medicine and Nursing Collection 2018 – NHS

Available at Anaesthesia from EBSCO (MEDLINE
Complete)

Abstract:

In aviation, the sterile cockpit rule prohibits non-essential
activities during critical phases of flight, takeoff and landing,
phases analogous to induction of, and emergence from,
anaesthesia. We studied distraction during 30 anaesthetic
inductions, maintenances and emergences. Mean (SD) noise
during emergence (58.3 (6.2) dB) was higher than during
induction (46.4 (4.3) dB) and maintenance (52 (4.5) dB;
p<0.001). Sudden loud noises, greater than 70 dB, occurred
more frequently at emergence (occurring 34 times) than at
induction (occurring nine times) or maintenance (occurring
13 times). The median (IQR [range]) of staff entrances or exits
were 0 (0-2 [0-7]), 6 (3-10 [1-18]) and 10 (5-12 [1-20]) for
induction, maintenance and emergence, respectively
(p<0.001). Conversations unrelated to the procedure occurred
in 28/30 (93%) emergences. These data demonstrate
increased distraction during emergence compared with
other phases of anaesthesia. Recognising and minimising
distraction should improve patient safety. Applying
aviation's sterile cockpit rule may be a useful addition to our
clinical practice.

Database: Medline

10. OPTIMIZING THE OPERATING THEATRE ENVIRONMENT

Author(s): Wong, Shing W; Smith, Richard; Crowe, Phil

Source: ANZ journal of surgery; Dec 2010; vol. 80 (no. 12);
p. 917-924

Publication Date: Dec 2010

Publication Type(s): Journal Article Review

PubMedID: 21114733

Available at ANZ journal of surgery - from Wiley Online Library Medicine and Nursing Collection 2018 - NHS

Abstract:

The operating theatre is a complex place. There are many potential factors which can interfere with surgery and predispose to errors. Optimizing the operating theatre environment can enhance surgeon performance, which can ultimately improve patient outcomes. These factors include the physical environment (such as noise and light), human factors (such as ergonomics), and surgeon-related factors (such as fatigue and stress). As individual factors, they may not affect surgical outcome but in combination, they may exert a significant influence. The evidence for some of these working environment factors are examined individually. Optimizing the operating environment may have a potentially more significant impact on overall surgical outcome than improving individual surgical skill.

Database: Medline

ADVOCACY

Healthcare doesn't serve advocates well.

The unspoken promise of unjust treatment is a well-worn reality.

This book could not have been written without first giving up work, and then my professional registration.

I have advocated on behalf of friends, colleagues and strangers all my nursing life and this book is merely the result of my learnings on their behalf.

For over thirty years, it has been my privilege to serve loyally the entire spectrum of the community, usually at the time of their greatest existential vulnerability.

I have been present untold times at the joy of birth, the heartbreak of death and at innumerable instances of misfortune in between.

In honour of my own humanity, I believe at this time it is my duty to make available this, my own work, for whatever assistance it may be.

Pete Smith

On this, the seventh hour of the sixth day of June, 2019

www.belowtenthousand.com

ABOUT THE AUTHOR

Pete Smith is just a guy at the shallow end of the gene pool.

He spent the first five years of his life under a farmhouse playing in the dirt with his Matchbox cars.

He spent the next eleven years surrounded by cows.

His brother, Greg, five years older, had severe Down Syndrome. Greg was much, much cooler than Pete could ever be.

So how did this impoverished kid who knew more about cows than humans end up as a career nurse?

And how did this unpolished introvert finish up co-creating what he calls 'the greatest thing in nursing since the Bristol Stool Chart'?

The world is a mysterious place.

Some would say complex, dangerous and chaotic.

But really, it is quite simple if we allow it to be.

In self-imposed exile from what he sees as the brutality of the healthcare system, Pete has a roof over his head, food in his belly, and now, back on the family farm, something to do each day.

He is unerringly accompanied in his work by his three-legged dog and, occasionally, by his three favourite people: his wife, son and daughter.

Lightning Source UK Ltd.
Milton Keynes UK
UKHW021434030720
365983UK00005B/732